Being Called to Care

Being Called to Care

Mary Ellen Lashley
Maggie T. Neal
Emily Todd Slunt
Louise M. Berman
and Francine H. Hultgren

Foreword by Peggy L. Chinn

State University of New York Press

Published by
State University of New York Press, Albany

For information, address State University of New York Press,
State University Plaza, Albany, N.Y. 12246

Production by M. R. Mulholland
Marketing by Theresa A. Swierzowski

Library of Congress Cataloging-in-Publication Data

Being called to care / Mary Ellen Lashley ... [et al.].
    p.   cm.
   Includes bibliographical references and index.
   ISBN 0-7914-1839-1 (HC : acid-free paper). -- ISBN 0-7914-1840-5
(PB : acid-free paper)
   1. Nursing--Philosophy.   2. Caring.   3. Vocation.   I. Lashley,
Mary Ellen, 1959–
RT84.5.B45   1994
610.73'01--dc20   93-7296
                                                               CIP

10 9 8 7 6 5 4 3 2 1

Contents

Foreword

I grew up the daughter of a minister. Almost daily, my parents spoke of "a call." Every major life decision involved waiting and listening for the call. Daily choices, both practical and ethical, were based on the call. The service provided to others was justified because of the call. Time and solitude were frequently sought and protected as valuable, necessary, if one were to hear the call. As a child trying to make sense of the world, "the call" formed a mystical image from which I formed structures of what is good, how it is to Be in the world, the meaning of service to others, the spiritual necessity of being in meaningful relation to others.

My childhood orientation to "the call," while rooted then in the structure of organized religion, grants me an understanding of the notion of "being called," and of what is called caring—an understanding that reaches far beyond the limits of any particular religious orientation. "Calling" can mean the power of naming. "A call" can mean the power of purpose. "Being called" can mean the existence that is signified by naming, as well as the fuel for action that is fired by purpose. "Called to care" is a willingness to Be in significant relation, to be responsive to others, to be in spirit together, in human existence together. In a deeply spiritual sense, it is the highest calling. In a profoundly practical sense, it is the most urgent calling beckoning all people on earth today.

Caring, a notion that is sometimes trivialized as merely something everyone can do, requiring little or no educational prowess, cannot be easily dismissed in a world that has been rendered spiritually bankrupt by a century of run-away technocratic materialism. Caring can be as exquisitely simple as a small act of kindness, or it can be as richly complex as the nurse skillfully bringing a premature infant and family through the first critical months to health, developmental wholeness, well positioned to develop as a sturdy child in a nurturing family. The human potential to care, like the human potential to be authentic, cannot be classified or characterized as a single "thing", nor can it conform to classifications. It cannot be boxed, packaged, or delivered on command. As a human potential, it can be envisioned, it can be imagined, it can be experienced, it can be learned, it can be nurtured. Caring can be called forth; it can be inspired. It can be called forth from any human. As a potential, it can be developed more fully as it is practiced, understood, responded to, explored, envisioned.

The important explorations and insights offered by the authors in this book provide vivid evidence of ways in which nurses exercise their responses to a call to care. This is not a sentimental text, nor is it a simple or singular approach. The text is not associated with religious ideology. It *is* deeply spiritual; it explores the common grounds of meaning in human existence. These authors have brought together insights that are grounded in nursing experience, transcend the limits of discrete moments of time and space, and offer for our consideration complex, difficult and challenging ideas and possibilities. For the student of caring, this book provides a rich resource for understanding the complex foundations upon which disciplined caring praxis rests. For the practitioner, this book provides a rich resource that can nurture the courage to act more fully, to hear more completely, to give voice to significant experience more confidently.

I commend the authors for their accomplishments represented in this work. I am confident that this work makes a significant contribution to the possibilities inherent in our potential as nurses, as people, to respond to the call to care.

Peggy L. Chinn, RN., Ph.D., F.A.A.N
Associate Dean for Academics
University of Colorado
School of Nursing

Acknowledgments

As a community of authors we are grateful for the opportunity to work together as colleagues and friends in the process of writing this book. We have encouraged and supported one another in special ways. As a result, our meetings fostered the lively conversations that made this book possible.

Our highest praise goes to the staff at SUNY Press. Lois G. Patton, Editor-in-Chief, believed in the possibilities we envisioned as we initially launched the book. Priscilla C. Ross, Editor, has strongly supported our efforts and provided ongoing direction for this project. We extend very special thanks to Megeen R. Mulholland, Production Editor, for being conscientious in providing editorial advice and in striving for the best possible book.

We acknowledge and thank the many students who shared their experiences and personal meanings that enabled us to gain new insights about the call to care and in our search for mutual understanding. Our deepest appreciation goes to the special students who participated in our dissertations for allowing their voices to be heard and for their contribution to our research.

Permission to reprint the following is gratefully acknowledged:

"Chapter XI" from *TAO TE CHING* by Lao Tsu, translated by Feng/English. Copyright © 1972 by Gia Fu-Feng and Jane English. Reprinted by permission of Alfred A. Knopf, Inc.

Comparison of Communitas and Social Structure, a table from "Imagining, changing, stabilizing: Maintaining momentum" by Louise M. Berman in *Toward a Renaissance of Humanity: Rethinking and Reorienting Curriculum and Instruction* (1988) edited by T. R. Carson and used with permission from Maxine Dunfee representing the World Council for Curriculum and Instruction.

Finally, our thanks to James R. Carpenter, Sara A. Lee, Sarah A. McCarthy, and Roberta A. Walsh for granting permission to include their stories, a poem, and the insightful reflections they wrote while completing courses with us.

Preface

Persons around the world share a sense of yearning, of caring, and of desiring wholeness. Although yearning for different or better ways of being is common to humankind, persons called into human service professions frequently feel the need to deal fully with their own meanings and longings so that they can be more fully present to others. Nurses, teachers, religious leaders, social workers, and concerned lay persons care. In fact they are constantly "being called to care." Thus the title of this book.

This book has three purposes. The first is to examine certain philosophical assumptions that underlie the call to care. As authors we have assumed that life in service with and to others is embedded in a need to be authentic, to acknowledge our vulnerabilities, and to live within the structures that bound our lives, at times seeking to reform the structures and at other times living amicably within them. Our assumptions have gone beyond our immediate worlds, for in our work as educators within human service professions we have found our students reflecting on these same assumptions and qualities.

Hence, a second purpose of this work is to make public several studies conducted with those preparing for entry to the service professions. Through interpretive inquiry, three of the authors worked with students who shared their meanings of becoming competent, of being with the elderly, and of being in a psychiatric nursing setting. In all of these studies issues of vulnerability, structure, and authenticity came forth as integral to being called to care.

Finally, a third purpose is to highlight insights, perspectives, and questions that persons interested in deepening their being called to care might want to consider within their work. What does it mean to dwell in a professional community? To create new possibilities?

This book is a collaborative effort among five persons, three of whom are nurse educators. The other two are broadly based curriculum theorists and researchers. All share an interest in interpretive inquiry. The studies reported are from nursing education; however, possible connections between nursing and other human service professionals are evident throughout the work. The ordering of the authors does *not* indicate the weight of the contribution to the volume. Each author assumed at different times different types of leadership.

The work contains many glimpses of teachers at work with students. We have tried to be reflective about our teaching and to uncover its richness for those involved, thus the chapters that follow show the many directions teaching can take.

For example, teaching may be face to face. In such cases, the teacher establishes a setting where a student may make sense of the world. Teaching may be side by side, as teacher and students make sense of text or other realia in the setting (Berman 1988b; Scudder & Mickunas 1985). Or, teaching may be a dance, as students and teacher move in and out of a circle, enriched by lively questions, fresh ideas, and new meanings of self.

As teachers and students encounter each other, knowledge, attitudes, values, longings, and desires may be shared. Occasionally, the teacher may lead the way, sharing wisdom and expertise. Ultimately, students lead the way, building upon the past and creating new meanings for self and the profession of which they are a part.

The authors in a sense engage in teaching with each other, sometimes face to face, as when we attempt to make meaning together, sometimes side by side, as when we read the texts of others or of those in a group. And sometimes, the teaching is in a circle dance as we celebrate having reached milestones in our thinking or writing.

The Authors

The authors come from four institutions of higher education in Maryland. Three of the writers are from nursing education but represent different institutions and different specialties. Mary Lashley is from Towson State University, where she teaches community health nursing. Maggie Neal teaches psychiatric nursing, interpretive inquiry, and curriculum theory at the University of Maryland at Baltimore. Emily Slunt is both an administrator and a professor of maternal-child-health nursing at Howard Community College. Louise Berman and Francine Hultgren are professors at the University of Maryland, College Park. Louise's field of study is curriculum theory and development, Francine's is home economics education, curriculum, interpretive and deconstructive inquiry.

All authors share an interest in rethinking, reshaping, and reinterpreting our fields. Sometimes gaps or overemphases are highlighted. Sometimes the heritage is valued, and at other times flaws in the heritage point out the need for political action. Sometimes, the necessity of new knowledge is seen. Our focus is on being called to care. Thus our discussion deals with questions and topics needing to be considered when the call to care is seen as integral to entering a profession, and sustaining the call is central to keeping one's personal and professional life dynamic.

What stimulated us to write the book? Perhaps it was the need to understand better our respective fields; or the desire to engage with others in sustained dialogue on such topics as caring, call, and teaching in helping professions; or the need to continue to consider "curriculum as Being." Perhaps it was a combination of the three. But even as we talked, wrote, and thought together, even as common threads seemed to hold us together, different skeins of interests and thoughts added variety to the tapestry we were weaving.

Mary is the youngest of the authors, having obtained advanced degrees in both nursing and education in fairly rapid succession. "Mastery of a knowledge community's normal discourse is the basic qualification for acceptance into that community" (Bruffee 1984, p. 643). Even as Mary was establishing herself as a nurse educator, she was trying to enter the broader community of education. In addition, she encountered professors who were talking about alternative educational perspectives, such as interpretive approaches to curriculum. These perspectives are not the dominant ones either in nursing or in colleges of education. Bruffee, building upon Rorty's concept of knowledge as social artifact calls knowledge-generating discourse "abnormal" discourse (p. 647). Thus, Mary was not only entering a school new to her but dealing with faculty who were setting aside the authority of traditional knowledge and searching for and attempting to build communities based upon different assumptions about persons and different goals for education. In a sense, as most researchers, she was dealing with her fields of study as abnormal discourse.

Mary frequently talks about vulnerability as she experiences the stress and loneliness of newness. She is asking new questions of life and turns to writers such as Frankl (1963) to answer the question: How does one experience suffering and yet find meaning in it?

Mary continues to contemplate the meanings of living in diverse communities. She thinks about being part of the community of nurse educators, where she is eager to maintain the rich heritage of nursing that shaped her thought. At the same time she thinks about providing opportunities where persons may change if they so desire. Education for Mary is not so much change in structure as change in people. In addition to sharing her own research "Being with the Elderly in Community Health Nursing" (Lashley 1989), Mary considers meanings of vulnerability in being called to care.

Maggie frequently talks about an interest in "structure," but not structure in a traditional sense. The term means to pile, build, assemble, and arrange. It comes from the same root as *heap* (Barnhart 1988, p. 1079). Although structure has connotations of conformity, Maggie's interpretations have intriguing twists that seem to suggest building something new out of the heap. She moves us toward a cultural analysis and understanding of structure. In addition to her expertise in nursing, Maggie is interested in the arts. As a hobby she makes stained glass lamps and other articles. Since she teaches psychiatric nursing, she explores different ways to bring artistry to teaching. In addition, Maggie describes herself as intuitive, as concerned with vision, as a risk taker, and as being present in the moment. Although she values long-range planning, Maggie sees planning as disempowering for her. Making the most of the present rather than planning for the future is what is most important to her.

Maggie in her teaching seeks to be as coequal with students as possible. Her desire to be present to and with students seems to create for some students epiphanies (Denzin 1989, pp. 15, 16), which are situations in which something comes to light, when there is a manifestation of the essential meaning of the essence of reality. She is concerned that students have deep, transformational experiences that help them see self and others in new, more meaningful ways.

Maggie contributes to this volume her considerations of structure in addition to her own research with nursing students. Her lines of inquiry deal with viewing students as works of art.

Emily ponders the meaning of authenticity in the various settings in which she finds herself. *Authentic* comes from a Greek word meaning "one who does a thing himself" (*Shorter Oxford*, 1968). Being genuine or bonafide is frequently equated with the term. Trustworthiness (Sisson 1966, p. 22) and acting on one's own authority (Barnhart 1988, p. 85) are integral to authenticity. What forms does authenticity take for the nurse educator? For the administrator? For the nurse? For a mother? For a wife? For a person who serves in a variety of capacities?

Emily raises questions relative to her own becoming. Although she may display different forms of being in the settings and functions of her life, she is constantly concerned about the central core of being— of *her* Being. She thoughtfully considers the meaning of the "call" to nursing.

Emily is not content to maintain the status quo in her life. In a sense she owns up to Caputo's consideration of authenticity as being in the flux and trying not to drown (Caputo 1987, p. 258). She continuously asks new questions and is committed to the notion of multiple lenses of knowing. She struggles with going beyond where she is—transcending—while still holding on to what she considers important.

Authenticity, for Emily, demands time for reflection, time for thinking, time for self-renewal. She appears to be searching for a way of being grounded in better ways of inhabiting the earth or a way of being ethical on her journey. In addition to dealing with the topic of authenticity, Emily shares her study on meanings nursing students have relative to becoming competent (Slunt 1989).

Louise is a long time inquirer into curriculum development. She is concerned about issues and topics that cut across education in a variety of kinds of settings. Thus she works with nurse educators, public and private school teachers and administrators, and other human service personnel. She attempts to understand the lived worlds of persons in their settings; therefore she has many transcultural and transnational concerns. At times, therefore, she dwells in settings that she feels she needs to understand better. In this way she feels she can converse with persons within the settings on problems of concern to them.

For example, when working with Emily, she wanted to deal more adequately with her questions about the clinical. Thus she spent time shadowing Emily in clinical experiences followed by conversations with her. She learned about the tough decisions nurse educators make as they live with nursing students and patients. She became aware of the many turns a call to care can take. In this work, Louise considers some of the broader meanings of being called to care. Her contributions to this volume resonate with the thoughts and concerns of those who see caring as foundational to curriculum development (Noddings 1992).

Francine, a student of hermeneutics, deconstruction, and other forms of interpretive inquiry, applies the philosophical underpinnings of such inquiry to her field of home economics. With others she has helped reconceptualize the field so that it has less emphasis upon the technical and more upon being and emancipatory interests for families. She consistently seeks to ask more penetrating questions, to peel back the layers of meaning of persons and their institutions, and to get at the essence of living. Her work in the transformation of home economics has had many implications for the transforming of nursing and nursing education. In this work she shares certain of her understandings of interpretive inquiry, using a deconstructive turn to illuminate a radical hermeneutics that reaches beyond Being.

All of the writers both individually and collectively ask questions about being called to care. All of the writers are concerned not only about theoretical issues, but also about the practical. Thus, the latter part of the work deals with creating new possibilities for caring. Attention is given to such topics as curriculum development, listening, centering, and questioning within caring communities.

At times, our voices may be heard singularly as persons report on meanings of experiences for them. When the study of one of the writers is reported, the first person may be used. Ordinarily one can tell from the context which of the authors is speaking. At other times, particularly the first and last chapters, the third person may predominate, as the reader is invited to share in our philosophical bases underlying our work or to consider our suggestions for curriculum or caring communities. The book is typical of lives in community, with a solo voice being heard at times and a chorus at others. After much deliberation, we decided the major author of each chapter should sign it.

Organization of the Text

Although the authors have followed a logical stucture in organizing the book, readers are invited to begin with chapters of most interest to them.

Part 1, "Setting the Context," opens with Louise's consideration in chapter 1, of the meaning of being called to care. In chapter 2, "Ways of Responding to the Call," Francine, through a deconstructive lens, considers what the response to a call might look like if one is guided by the claims of natural, universal, or rational inquiry (empiricism, hermeneutics, or critical social theory). For some, Francine's chapter may be useful grounding in emerging schools of philosophical thought. Others may prefer to read about concrete practices first and later return to theoretical grounding.

Part 2, "Living the Call as Inquiring Learners," contains experiences of living the call as inquirers, teachers, and learners. The experiences were those described in the process of gathering text for doctoral research. Small groups of nursing students in two baccalaureate programs and one associate degree program participated in the research studies. They shared meaningful experiences regarding their nursing education experiences with a particular focus on the practice arena. Being with patients in acute care, psychiatric and community based settings provided the opportunity for dialogue and reflection. Personal meanings were explored as both the learners and inquirers sought to understand at a deeper level. Three common themes are explored: in chapter 3, Mary explores vulnerability; in chapter 4, Emily deals with authenticity; and in chapter 5, Maggie treats issues of structure. These common threads are viewed as central to the call to care.

Part 3, "Experiencing the Call through Stories in Nursing and Education," includes individual accounts of the three studies originally prepared as doctoral dissertations. Through phenomenological perspectives, different contexts in which the call to care in nursing may be lived out were considered. In chapter 6, Mary writes about being with the elderly. Chapter 7 contains Emily's experiences with her students as they become competent in nursing. And in chapter 8 Maggie writes about the student as a work of art.

Part 4, "Sustaining the Call though Being in Possibility," contains three chapters. In chapter 9, "Curricular Challenges," Louise considers reflection, writing, storytelling, and metaphor as alternative approaches in assisting people in finding meaning within their experiences. In chapter 10, Francine invites us to pose a new question as to who is at the center of being called. Her chapter is titled "Being Called to Care—or—Caring Being Called to Be: Do We Have a New Question?" The final chapter focuses on "Keeping the Call Alive" in which listening, centeredness, and community are considered as central to sustaining the call.

This project is a natural outgrowth of lived experiences and journeys. For Mary, Emily, and Maggie the experience was conducting and completing dissertations—journeys taken in the presence of caring others, especially Louise and Francine. The journeys have changed our lives forever. Through deconstructive lenses, three significant themes that repeatedly appeared in our pedagogy with students and within our own place of call were revealed. Our inquiry about the themes—vulnerability, authenticity and structure/conformity gave rise to this project.

Reverby (1987) contends that the contemporary problems faced by caregivers are rooted in historical obligations to care in a culture that does not value caring. Rather than responding to specific issues about the "order to care," our inquiry centers on something more fundamental—the call itself that resonates in each student and within our own lives. This call is often forgotten in the busyness or obligations of daily practice yet clearly remains an issue in our lives. It is the reason for our being who we are. After addressing the more fundamental issues, we return to question our response to the call within technical structures that often do not support our authentic being with others and the vulnerability created as we attempt to transform our places of call into hospitable dwelling places.

Louise M. Berman

References

Barnhart, R. K. (Ed.). (1988). *The Barnhart dictionary of etymology.* Bronx: H. W. Wilson.

Berman, L. M. (1988a). Dilemmas in teaching caring: An "outsider's" perspective. *Nursing Connections, 1*(3), 5–15.

Berman, L. M. (1988b). Face-to-face or side-by-side: Teaching graduate courses in curriculum. *Teaching Education, 2*(2), 84–87.

Bruffee, K. A. (1984). Collaborative learning and the "conversation of mankind." *College English, 46*(7), 635–52.

Caputo, J. D. (1987). *Radical hermeneutics: Repetition, deconstruction, and the hermeneutic project.* Bloomington: Indiana University Press.

Denzin, N. K. (1989). *Interpretive interactionism.* Newbury Park, CA: Sage.

Frankl, V. E. (1955, 1963). *Man's search for meaning: An introduction to logotheraphy* (rev. ed.) (Ilse Lach, Trans.). New York: Washington Square Press. (Original work published 1946)

Lashley, M. (1989). Being with the elderly in community health nursing: Exploring lived experience through reflective dialogue (Doctoral dissertation. University of Maryland, College Park). *Dissertation Abstracts International, 51,* 729A.

Noddings, N. (1992). *The challenge to care in schools: An alternative approach to education.* New York: Teachers College Press.

Reverby, S. (1987). *Ordered to care: The dilemma of American nursing.* New York: Cambridge University Press.

Roget's II: The new thesaurus. (1980). Boston: Houghton Mifflin.

Scudder, J. R., & Mickunas, A. (1985). *Meaning, dialogue, and enculturation: Phenomenological Philosophy of Education.* Lanham, MD: University Press.

The shorter Oxford English dictionary. (1968). (3rd ed.). Oxford: Clarendon Press.

Sisson, A. F. (1966). *Sisson's word and expression locator.* West Nyack, NY: Parker.

Slunt, E. T. (1989). Becoming competent: A phenomenological inquiry into its meaning by nursing students. (Doctoral dissertation, University of Maryland, College Park). *Dissertation Abstracts International, 51,* 1196B.

Webster's new dictionary of synonyms. (1984). Springfield, MA: Merriam-Webster.

I

Setting the Context

Human service professionals, and indeed people in general, frequently talk about being called—and in the case of the authors of this book being called to care. In this section, Louise and Francine examine the title of this book and the methods of thinking and inquiring that guide our work.

In chapter 1, Louise explores three fundamental questions: What does it mean to be called? What does it mean to sustain a call? What does it mean to be called to care? Drawing upon insights of the authors of the subsequent chapters, as well as those of philosophers, theologians, and human service professionals, Louise creates a framework for thinking about the questions and issues predominant in this work.

In chapter 2, Francine directs attention to emerging philosophical schools of thought and the parts they play in shaping responses to the call to care. She deals with the varieties of postmodern thinking and their contributions in framing responses to being called to care.

1

What Does It Mean to Be Called to Care?

Louise M. Berman

As we authors gathered around the table to reflect upon the meaning of being called to care we shared a variety of insights in response to the question: What does it mean to you to be called to care? Here are just a few snippets from our conversations.

Emily: I can remember when I took aptitude tests in high school testing very high in science and very high in the social area—wanting to work with people. The tests affirmed what I was already thinking. I had done volunteer work. Nursing was the profession I wanted to enter. Interest in people and interest in science seemed to go together. I find these two to be a constant thread in my work and in my studies...I think both of these contribute to the feeling of being called...I wanted to contribute to society in a different way, beyond my own family, although my family certainly has been central in my life...There is a certain spiritual sense that goes along with being called. Both the call and the sustaining of the call have a spiritual component to them.

Maggie: I think that for me the call to care was the commitment that grew out of family life, of needing to be responsible in many ways, of having an organized structured family life focused around education, around religion, where I saw parents making a commitment to working with and taking care of people. Sometimes we even took people into our home. I think my original response to the notion of calling and caring emerged from that...In psychiatric nursing you listen *with* heart. You are not needing to know what is going on under the skin except as you do it with dialogue.

Francine: I think one of the things I observe in working with students
              becoming teachers is that their sense of care is like a caring
              for, a doing *for* others...One of the elements of living out
              care in my own work is the sense of relation that you
              establish with one another in that caring relationship or in
              that being with one another in a caring way...Coupled with
              that relational aspect, of caring, I think is the claim made
              on you by somebody else...I think my own professional
              attention to caring came with Huebner's work (1987), which
              says that as you develop the vocation of being a teacher, it
              is that sense of living out your daily life as a way of being.

Mary: Is a calling an event, a way of being, or a response? Initially
              I came to the conclusion that it was a way of being, and then
              I thought of the notion of response. I do think that a calling
              is a response. It is that which compels us to move our life
              in a certain direction, to make choices and to live out our
              lives in meaningful ways. It might be a response to someone
              or something, but then it must be a response to
              persons...the primacy of the person, the face of the other
              is fundamental to the call...In a sense we are all willed or
              called to be in communion with others.

Louise: A telephone rings. An unknown and unexpected voice
              offers a position. An affirmative response is given...Eight
              years later another telephone call. Another unanticipated
              voice offers a position. Another affirmative response...The
              calls mentioned were significant in that I had an interior
              readiness to accept the invitations extended to me. In a sense
              the calls got to the essence of my being, perhaps because
              of the challenges, values, and possibilities inherent in the
              calls...My calling is to be with persons from varieties of
              educational settings. These persons are concerned with
              developing, changing, studying or interpreting curriculum
              in the settings of which they are part. My calling intersected
              with the callings of Maggie, Emily, and Mary, professors of
              nursing, as together we thought about ways of being and
              teaching in schools of nursing. Thus when a call came from
              one of the nurse educators to begin to think with them about
              a book, my reaction was to join them. Such an experience
              is in line with the values, predispositions, and attitudes
              which underlie my call and keep it in perspective.[1]

The windows on conversations among us as authors caused a
realization that being called has many dimensions. Furthermore, we

found that each of us highlights different concepts of being called. We see that although for some, being called has some clear decisions points or breaks in our lives, for all of us the sustaining of the call has a claim upon us as we dwell within communities that nurture that call.

The remainder of this chapter then deals with three interrelated questions. What does it mean to be called? What does it mean to sustain the call? What does it mean to be called to care?

What Does It Mean To Be Called?

How easy it would be if we could program calls for persons! If such were possible, a national agency might keep track of career and professional trends, and institutions could prepare individuals to fill necessary slots. Such does not ordinarily happen in a democracy where individual choice undergirds much critical decision making.

In the United States, despite freedom to choose at an individual level, persons have unequal access to resources and ideas affecting their professional decision making. Racial, socioeconomic, ethnic, gender, and other inequities have a bearing upon access to information, role models, and knowledge bases that might influence professional career choices. In other instances the mores or traditions of one's peer group may influence one's call toward a career choice. Directions may not be clearly established when choices are made. Some may embark on a path without a map, without a sense of direction, but move into a call after they have begun a profession.

For example, Mary said:

I'll have to confess that I never did feel called into nursing. I feel like I fell into nursing. I think it had a lot to do with life experiences and situations, social contexts that I was embedded in at the time. I had the opportunity to have some work experiences in a hospital setting that oriented me to nursing. I had choices to make in college. I really didn't know what I wanted to do with my life. That was something I was familiar with. It was more comfortable and less threatening to enter into. As I learned more about nursing, as I got into the profession, I grew into it. I grew to love it, but I definitely did not feel called from the very beginning.

Emily talked about having aptitudes in science and working with people. This self-knowledge pointed her toward striving to enhance the quality of persons' lives through a healthier way of being. The direction was deliberate and planned and seemed right. "I have always felt that I have one life to live. I need to use my talents to the maximum that I can within that time period."

Although both Mary and Emily suggested different modes of decision making relative to entrance to nursing, both have sustained that entry-level decision in significant ways. Thus, call comes in a variety of ways.

As we explore the question of what it means to be called, particularly to human service, we find some partial responses to the question. Being called may come about as *restlessness* of spirit, from feelings of indecision, from being at transitional periods in life, or from a sense of longing, desire, yearning, or wonder. Sometimes these inner strivings are voiced, other times they may be hidden beneath the busyness of life, or they may take the form of wanting to do *for* others (Francine). Or that restlessness may take the form of feeling one needs to acquire knowledge in order to carry out certain humane ends.

At times the call may be very direct. Witness the biblical stories of Samuel in the temple or Jesus' calls to his disciples. The call may be so direct that it comes via telephone, letters, or today by fax. Certainly all invitations are not necessarily calls. The person receiving the message needs to have an inward receptivity to act upon it.

Call may be an awakening to a sense of purpose for our lives. "It can involve an accelerating sense of inner direction. It can emerge through a gnawing feeling that we need to do a specific thing" (Farnham et al. 1991, p. 7).

Call requires that we take responsibility for using the building blocks given to us—"intelligence, creativity, sensitivity, love"—and see what can be done with them (Farnham et al. 1991, p. 14). Our innate faculties are guided by knowledge and embedded in our sense of caring for our fellow travelers. The initial call may make us feel anxious—even anguished—vulnerable, and at risk. But a sense of call is invitational to probing into the knowledge bases of the community or professional arena.

The diligent search into knowledge is undergirded by a call to the face of the other in "inter-human relationship" (Levinas 1985, p. 97). "The face orders and ordains me" (1985 p. 97). The face of the other in suffering or wellness is what calls, claims, and calms human restlessness. Faces that make claims on us may change, the surges of restlessness may come and go. But it is that entrance to the call that opens up a way of being, a sacred trust, a continuous yearning to sustain the call. We learn to "be comfortable with reasonable doubt, openness, and unsureness if we are to respond afresh to that which is given us afresh" (Huebner 1987, p. 25).

In summary, a call ordinarily involves one speaking, one listening, and a response. That speaking and listening may be figurative, but an inner dialogue takes place that eventuates in a response. A call involves hearing and reflecting upon experiences in one's history and deciding upon next steps. It means an intentional living of life and continuous decision making in line with one's intentions. A call may be considered an *evocation*, which is a calling forth or the opportunity to enter new possibilities, to ask new questions, to be with others in new ways, or to become more conscious—to notice what was taken for granted. Indeed, a call may be subtle, or it may resound as a trumpet.

A call may also be a benediction (meaning speaking well). Thus, those who feel a call may speak in such a way that well-being is promoted. The speaking comes from a self that is authentic because it may have taken time to uncover or create a call, to nurture it, and to reflect upon it.

The creation or uncovering of a call may result in an epiphany or a transformational experience (Denzin 1989, p. 15). A new kind of reality may emerge as a result of a turning point. Passion, direction, and a sense of well-being may characterize an epiphany.

Indeed, a call is a heightened response to our human restlessness.

What Does It Mean to Sustain the Call?

Each day brings fresh ideas, fresh challenges, and fresh ways of seeing the world. The regularities, and surprises are what invite us to sustain a call. We live each day in risk, responsibility, and responsiveness.

Risk taking is what propels us into uncharted waters. Risk invites us to make intuitive leaps in our imaginations and to act upon our hunches. The more skilled the individual the more possibility for making intuitive leaps, for the experienced person has skills and knowledges not yet attained by the novice. In a sense, risk invites an openness to the mysteries of the day.

It is the sense of responsibility that helps sustain the call. Responsibility invites us to an "accelerating sense of inner direction" (Farnham et al. 1991, p. 7). As individuals assume more responsibility for centering and renewing the self, they are more able to work in tandem with others, whether they may be doctors, nurses, social workers, or patients.

Responsibility means increasing one's skills in discernment. Discernment is a sensitive blend of observational, analytical, and normative skills that allow what is hidden to emerge. It is wisdom in the midst of complexity, meaning finding in the absence of hope, and clarity in the valley of shadows. The linear development of skills and knowledge is an anathema to discernment unless individuals have learned to relate such skills and knowledge to larger wholes, including the call to nursing.[2]

Responsibility to the human service worker then means tuning into the call of the other for understanding of his or her own pain and suffering. Pain has different meanings to different people in different cultures (Morris 1991). How does the person in the immediate setting see and feel his or her pain? What are the mores relative to pain and suffering within the culture of which the individual is part?[3]   •

Being called assumes an ongoingness and responsiveness. The telephone does not ring once. It rings frequently. The call comes in the moment and evokes a presentness. Subsequent calls, however, may mean a revitalizing and a renewing and probably a reconstituting of the initial commitment. We are called by different people, to different contexts, and in different times. Sustaining the call involves my response to my initial commitment in different configurations of space, in different periods of time, and with different kinds of persons.

Sustaining the call also has a qualitative aspect. The quality of being called involves listening and speaking. It involves being attuned to others—in the case of nursing, the patient, the doctor, other health professionals, and family members. In a sense, the quality of sustaining the call can be likened to sensitivity jazz musicians bring to those with whom they are playing.

A nursing student offers other musical metaphors to enhance understanding of the quality of being called. Regina writes:

> In the song of health care, the nurse is the harmonizer. To be part of the singing, however, the nurse must be aware of his/her own voice. Is he/she an alto, soprano, bass, tenor? What is his/her range, what octaves are beyond him/her, what key is he/she most strong in? He/she listen to the voice of the client, note by note with the client, but still a distinct voice. One note up, together up. One octave down, the nurse maintains the harmony to help the client. In harmonizing, the nurse takes into account the rhythm composed by the doctor and also keeps in beat with other health professionals' input. And so the nurse listens to the client's voice, the silent rests of the client's voice, the flatness of the client's voice—all a part of the nurse's tuning into the client's individual song. The nurse is to harmonize, to bring out the distinct quality of the client's voice and provide them with a melodious guide

to sing with others. . .Music lessons are discipline for the nurse. But he/she must sing his/her own song with help from others and alone. (Neal 1989, pp. 121–22)

Quality involves understanding nuance, "eloquence, wit, grace, and economy" (Kronenberger 1969, p. 170). The quality of being called is dependent upon the creation and re-creation of vision, appreciation of the complexity of the call, and wisdom and courage in meeting the challenges of the call. The initial call to care differs from later calls to care in that more experienced persons have a fuller grasp of the meaning of quality in being called to care (Benner 1984).

So what is the essence of being called to care?

What Does It Mean to Be Called to Care?

Being called and sustaining a call have active as well as reflective qualities. Calls sometimes come with loud knocks, other times with inner or still small voices. Changes frequently follow calls, particularly as persons enter transitional periods, move forward with others in community, and find themselves in periods of growth.

If we try to untangle the essence of being called to care we find that there are no hierarchically or chronologically arranged concepts. The essence of being called to care is in *response*, as Mary says, each response being contingent on understanding persons and their contexts.

Here are some possible ways to think about one's self and others as one struggles with meanings of the call to care.

Finding one's self. Throughout this work notions of authenticity and vulnerability surface as consideration is given to being with others. But what kind of a being enters into a relationship with others? As one finds personal wholeness both through self-reflection—sometimes anguish (Pritzkau 1970, p. 10)—and through being with others, one is better able to enter into healing relationships with others. Finding one's self is not something that is done once and for all. Rather, it is a constant response to an inner summons. It is self-renewal. It is feeling centered. Thus, being called to care has a major component of self-caring—of owning up to shortcomings (Caputo 1987, p. 59) and yet having the impetus and desire to "live out our historical lives" (1987, p. 258). In a sense, finding one's self is a search for authenticity—a wading into the flux and trying not to drown (1987, p. 258).

"In following a calling a person follows an invitation to embark on a journey to selfhood. A calling is discovered; it evolves and is a way of life, a way of being with others" (Slunt 1989, p. 81). In a sense, being centered is essential if one is to focus and to establish communion with others (Savary & Berne 1988, p. 24) . Centering is a holistic process, involving body, mind, and spirit, in which persons are present to themselves.

Although finding one's self has a reflective component, it paradoxically may take place in the company of and in communication with others. Thus, being called to care invites us to be with others. We are called to focus on the other—to see not only persons but the face of the other.

Seeing the face of the other. In a sense, the face is the threshold to another's being. The face may beckon, make a claim on us. When we see the face, it may invite us into its being. At the threshold the door may be partially ajar, beckoning us to come to enter, to come to know the person more fully. According to Beittel with Beittel (1991), "Doors connect with thresholds, and ever since ancient times thresholds have been considered sacred" (p. 84). When we really see the face of the other, we are accepting our most basic mode of responsibility. "I owe more to the other than to myself" (Kearney 1984, pp. 59–60).

When we enter the threshold of the other, or see the face of the other, we respond in an ethical manner: "access to the face is straightaway ethical. You turn yourself to the other as toward an object when you see a nose, eyes, a forehead, a chin, and you can describe them. The best way of encountering the other is not even to notice the color of his eyes! When one observes the color of the eyes, one is not in social relationship with the other" (Levinas 1985, p. 85).

Since those of us in human service professions are so tuned in to being careful observers of external signs, Levinas's caution to respond to the face permits a way of being that opens doors to an indwelling with the person.

Entering into. Being called to care means having a voice and entering into relationships with the other—sharing the joys, fears, and darkness of others. When I enter into the world of others, I meet the other in weakness of body but possibly strength of spirit, in fears but also in joy, in apprehension but also in faith. Life at best for most persons is full of paradoxes and contradictions. My task is to see the other face to face and to permit myself to experience that face, occasionally allowing for ruptures in my thinking as the face of the other challenges me to responsiveness and responsibility.

Suffering with. Nouwen talks about care coming from a root, meaning "lament" (1974, p. 34). In her discussion of care, Emily talks about two threads—the one has to do with being troubled and anxious for and with another, the other with the actions generated as a feeling of responsiveness to and responsibility for the other (Slunt 1989, pp. 39, 40). Thus, being called to care means stepping into the anguish of the other and simultaneously suffering with the other. At the same time the nurse is mobilizing ethical and intellectual energies to reflect on *more* than suffering. Nursing and other human service professions are called upon to engage in paradoxical, compelling, and contradictory feeling and actions as they suffer with others. They do not have the luxury of being immobilized. Being is called forth that is both suffering with the other and at the same time transcending the present state of the other.

Becoming one with. Despite the complexity of being called to deal with multiple realities, one is also called to be one with others, to commune. The nurse may feel a deep-seated concern for the being of the other (Lashley 1989, p. 6). Such may mean that one sees through the lenses of the other or steps out of one's own frame of reference into that of the other. Noddings (1984) talks about "engrossment." The person enters the world of the other. Individuals "feel" with the other (Neal 1989, p. 45).

Responding to. Pain, frustration, and possibly uncertainty may bond patient and nurse in a symmetrical relationship. They see each other face to face. On the other hand, the nurse may be in an asymmetrical relation to the patient as she responds to his exigencies. The nurse may respond by:

- dwelling with—watching the patient, being observant, giving protection, listening to
- creating structure—establishing ways to see that necessary tasks associated with the patient's well-being are accomplished
- giving voice—dealing with the particular knowledge and skill appropriate to the context
- being patient with institutional imperfections—handling constraints, contingencies and dilemmas with wisdom
- sharing knowledge, information, and insights that help the patient understand his or her own situation
- extending being through the use of the hand—touching, mediating between technology and the person
- standing beside—encouraging the person to go on
- standing behind—taking the lead from the patient

Hoping with. In times of crisis, seeming abandonment, the nurse is in a "privileged in-between position to foster the good of the patient" (Bishop & Scudder 1990, p. 140). Being in-between means decisions may be based upon a moral sense, a sense of hope for the patient. Emily talks about balancing the pain with hopefulness (Slunt 1989, p. 184).

Reflecting upon. Each encounter with another invites reflection on the way one responds to the call to care. Reflecting upon involves consideration of one's own humanity, one's response to the other, and one's ways of envisioning fresh possibilities. Creative reflection involves transformation of the self by the self (Nozick 1990, p. 39). As I reflect upon my experiences with others, I may obtain new insights about myself, thus enabling me to see others with fresh understandings.

Being called to care involves a rethinking of what it means to be in places and spaces where anxiety, dilemmas, and hurt abound. It means not so much revolutionizing nursing or other caregiving professions as it does uncovering aspects of the profession that have been taken for granted, questioning what is historically grounded or tradition bounded and reconstructing perspectives on nursing or other human service professions.

In this work, three major themes integral to being called to care are considered. The first, authenticity has to do with the wholeness and genuineness of the person. It also is the experience "in which one has present awareness about [self] in relation to...surroundings" (Pritzkau 1970, p. 1). Emily considers the meaning of authenticity for those reexamining nursing. Vulnerability, the second theme, suggests an openness or potential for harm, according to Mary. Such is essential if true healing is to take place. Vulnerability and authenticity suggest personal attributes necessary to the transformation of nursing practice. Maggie treats a third theme, structure, referring to the framework central to dealing with and organizing knowledge or experience. Thus, the authentic and vulnerable person works within a framework which enriches the call to care. Each of these themes is considered as we move through the book. But first we consider ways of responding to the call as seen through different philosophical lenses.

Notes

1. Prior to writing this chapter, I tape recorded individual conversations with the authors and transcribed them. We talked about some of the underpinnings of this text—what a call means, what caring means, and other topics pertinent to the text.

2. For a useful discussion of discernment see Farnham et al. (1991).

3. For a consideration of diversity of experiences and expressions in patients' dealing with pain and suffering, see Morris (1991).

References

Beittel, K., with Beittel, J. (1991). *A celebration of art and consciousness.* State College, PA: Happy Valley Healing Arts.

Benner, P. (1984). *From novice to expert: Excellence and power in clinical nursing practice.* Menlo Park, CA: Addison-Wesley.

Bishop, A. H., & Scudder, J. R., Jr. (1990). *The practical, moral, and personal sense of nursing: A phenomenological philosophy of practice.* Albany: State University of New York Press.

Caputo, J. D. (1987). *Radical hermeneutics: Repetition, deconstruction, and the hermeneutic project.* Bloomington: Indiana University Press.

Denzin, N. K. (1989). *Interpretive interactionism.* Newbury Park, CA: Sage.

Farnham, S. G., Gill, J. P., McLean, R. T., & Ward, S. M. (1991). *Listening hearts.* Harrisburg, PA: Morehouse.

Huebner, D. (1987). The vocation of teaching. In F. S. Bolin & J. M. Falk (Eds.), *Teacher renewal: Professional issues, personal choices* (pp. 17–29). New York: Teachers College Press.

Kearney, R. (1984). *Dialogues with contemporary continental thinkers: The phenomenological heritage.* Dover, NH: Manchester University Press.

Kronenberger, L., (Ed.). (1969). *Quality: Its image in the arts.* New York: Atheneum.

Lashley, M. (1989). Being with the elderly in community health nursing: Exploring lived experience through reflective dialogue. (Doctoral dissertation, University of Maryland, College Park). *Dissertation Abstracts International, 51,* 729A.

Levinas, E. (1985). *Ethics and infinity. Conversations with P. Nemo* (R. A. Cohen, Trans.). Pittsburgh: Duquesne University Press.

Morris, D. (1991). *The culture of pain.* Berkeley: University of California Press.

Neal, M. T. (1989). A room with a view: Uncovering the essence of student experience in a clinical nursing setting (Doctoral dissertation, University of Maryland, College Park). *Dissertation Abstracts International, 50,* 2847B.

Noddings, N. (1984). *Caring: A feminine approach to ethics and moral education.* Berkeley: University of California Press.

Nouwen, H. J. M. (1974). *Out of solitude.* Notre Dame: Ave Maria Press.

Nozick, R. (1989, 1990). *The examined life: Philosophical reflections.* New York: Simon & Schuster.

Pritzkau, P. T. (1970). *On education for the authentic.* Scranton: International Textbook Company.

Savary, L. M., & Berne, P. H. (1988). *Kything: The art of spiritual presence.* New York: Paulist Press.

Slunt, E. T. (1989). Becoming competent: A phenomenological inquiry into its meaning by nursing students (Doctoral dissertation. University of Maryland, College Park). *Dissertation Abstracts International, 51,* 1196B.

2

Ways of Responding to the Call

Francine H. Hultgren

To be called is to have a sense of responsibility and obligation, to be answerable—in short, one way to look at it is to have a vocation (Huebner 1987). If we look at our response to the call to care, the subject of this book, we must address the question of the ways in which we might answer the call, or as Caputo puts it, "to hear what is calling in the call" (1988, p. 61). We cannot merely respond to the call but must assume responsibility for it—to hold it in question and question our continual ability to respond. As Caputo says, "The height of responsibility is to wonder about the *origin* of what calls for a response" (1988, p. 64). This chapter reflects some wonderings about possible responses to the call to care that grow out of different philosophical orientations, so that we might be more attentive to the call of the calling that is caring. Subsequent chapters reflect examples of these orientations and questioning.

Origin of the Call: Living in the Tension Between Technological Determination and the Search for Being

Working together as a group of educators with backgrounds in nursing, curriculum, and home economics, we have been caught by a similar tension that seems to be lived out in our professional lives: between technological determination and the search for Being, or as we have described it, "the call to care." The following concern about the image of nursing has been expressed by Maggie, Emily, Mary, and the students with whom they work: Nursing is more than caring and nurturance, but nursing is not recognized for its rich knowledge base. As much as caring is central, it is not looked at as being as important as the knowledge base; maybe even more telling is the absence of care in the knowledge base itself. Who determines the *is* and the *more than?*

Coming from a field that has also been technically determined, home economics, Francine asks: What's it like to live in your own metaphor, as opposed to somebody else's imposition? (Berman, Hultgren, Lee, Rivkin, & Roderick 1991). Emily posits similar questions in her dissertation: What has the image of the nurse allowed the nurse to be? What kinds of tensions arise from the contradictions in the call, the image and the reality? (Slunt 1989).

A second element of this tension has to do with language, as acknowledged by Louise, wherein she asks: What kinds of language facilitate the issues inherent in the dialectic in which most persons abide? (Berman, Hultgren, Lee, Rivkin, & Roderick 1991). Emily says: I recognize the need to immerse myself in the new language of Being as a means to reduce the tension or weight of the technical language I bring (Slunt 1987). Maggie questions: What is it like to change your focus?—To go beyond the concise technical clinical terminology of nursing? How do you break out of a place in which you have been encapsulated? (Neal 1987). But in the rush to leave the technical paradigm, there is a looking back over the shoulder as Mary wonders: "How can I inspire students to push beyond the limitations of their present perspectives without negating or ignoring the inherent worth of their personal history?" (Lashley 1990, p. 1). Emily also acknowledges: I recognize that I cannot throw off the technocratic; I can see some value to aspects of it (Slunt 1987).

In light of these tensions that we continue to experience as educators, we surfaced the following questions:

- How do we as humans come to understand ourselves?
- How does technology and a technological determination affect this process?
- What kind of people do we want to be as we live with technology?

The origin of what calls for a response to these questions has to do with tension between the technological and our search for meaning through Being. Heidegger's *The Question Concerning Technology* (1977) is helpful in this struggle; he suggests the need to reconsider the necessity of preparing a free relationship to technology—to see it as a way of revealing, rather than something to be merely controlled. As Heidegger says, we must catch sight of what comes to presence in technology instead of merely staring at the technological.

One way of looking at our response to the call to care arising from this technological tension might be through the different stances we would take if we were guided by the claims of natural, universal, or rational modes of inquiry (i.e., empiricism, hermeneutics, or critical social theory) with their respective representative principles/interests of control/prediction, being/understanding, and reason/emancipation. While we choose these different paradigms for purposes of contrast and continued questioning, we along with Lather (1991) are careful to bear in mind what Atkinson, Delamont and Hammersley (1988) say about conceptual frameworks: "Classifying research and researchers into neatly segregated 'paradigms' or 'traditions' does not reflect the untidy realities of real scholars...and may become an end in itself...'Traditions' must be treated not as clearly defined, real entities but only as loose frameworks for dividing research" (p. 243).

As Lather (1991) suggests, paradigms might be considered useful transitional concepts to help us move toward a more adequate human science. We seek such a movement here as we attempt to illuminate the potential contribution of a radical hermeneutics (Caputo 1987), which seeks a collaboration between hermeneutics and deconstruction. To accomplish our examination/questioning of these different responses to the call to care, it would seem that deconstruction has something to offer us, since the project of deconstruction is described as a vocation—a response to a call. As Derrida says, "deconstruction is, in itself, a positive response to an alterity which necessarily calls, summons or motivates it" (Kearney 1984, p. 118).

An alterity is described as otherness and absence of meaning or self (Margolis 1985). As we use a deconstructive gaze to consider what is absent in the various ways we might respond to the call to care, the following question might serve to focus our gaze: *What has been excluded by what calls itself care?* In pursuit of that question, we might become more sensitive to the texture and meaning of care in our lives as nurses and educators and heed Aoki's (1991) urging: "Time-honored words...with their frozen meanings need to be placed into turbulence, alert to the multiplicity of meanings and, as well, to the legitimation and delegitimation of certain of these meanings" (p. ii).

Dimensions for Understanding the Responsibility/Response-ability of Deconstruction in the Discourse and Practice of Care

"Professions are constituted by what is said and done in their name. Regularities in what is said (discourse) and done (practice) are based on shared beliefs and values ranging across tasks accomplished, problems addressed, values articulated, and research undertaken" (Cherryholmes 1988, p. 1).

Deconstruction, in the Derridean sense, concerns itself with the laying bare of how discourse is constructed, showing how a discursive system functions, including what it excludes or denies (Pinar & Reynolds 1992). It is also a political activity that exposes the ideological function and content of discursive systems. To look at the discourse and practice of care in the professions of nursing and education through a deconstructive lens is to call into question the meaning it has acquired in different social and institutional contexts and to disrupt some of the binary oppositions (autonomy/nurturance, reason/emotion, public/private, right/duty, love/labor) that have served to reinforce the power dualities in the gendered construction of caring (Abel & Nelson 1990).

The work of deconstruction is to keep the ruling discourse in question, and as such it is ongoing, always unfinished work: not a position, but a praxis; not a theoretical outlook, but an activity (Caputo 1987). To that end it seeks liberation from all oppressive, regularizing, normalizing, and exclusionary discourses. In the words of Caputo, deconstruction is an un-doing, a kind of *"Ab-bauen,"* which does not raze but releases: " *'Ab-bau'* means a dismantling or undoing of a surface apparatus which has been allowed to build up over an originary experience—a dismantling not in order to level but in order to retrieve. Its function then is positive, to break through the encrusted in order to recover the living experience, which has since grown old and stiff" (1987, p. 64). It is not the intent of this chapter to provide a comprehensive analysis of postmodern thought; however, to understand the work of deconstruction, it is necessary to see its link to structuralism and poststructuralism.

Postmodernism, also called modernity, is characterized by a crisis in legitimation, specifically of knowledge, wherein there is an attitude of suspicion or lack of belief that prevails in relation to master narratives (overarching philosophies) (Lyotard 1989; Martusewicz 1992). It is a response to modernism's goal for philosophy of achieving a basic, fundamental knowledge or a seeking of grounds that will allow for certainty in knowledge. Assumptions about what constitutes knowledge or the very possibility of knowing have been placed deeply into question. Structuralism, a multifaceted movement of major importance to postmodernism, rejects the notion of a unified knowing subject and adopts the notion of knowledge and subjectivity as inscribed in culture through language. As Martusewicz (1992) defines it, "structuralism is based on the assumption that social and cultural phenomena are more than simply material phenomena. Human actions and events have meaning and, moreover, are dependent upon an underlying system of relations and distinctions that make meaning possible and define the form that such actions and events may take" (p. 132).

As a major contributor to structuralist thought, Levi-Stauss (1972) promotes the notion that functional oppositions produce meaning in a society, wherein binary oppositions such as objective/subjective, man/woman, light/dark come to have meaning because of the structural differences between them. The word valued by the structure is stated first and the disvalued word second. The origin of meaning, then, is found not in the author of the discourse (as in phenomenology) but in language itself. Meaning is located in structures, not in individuals, as the subject is decentered and emphasis is given to structured relationships.

Poststructuralist thought grew out of the claim that structuralist analyses are caught up in the processes and mechanisms they are analyzing (Culler 1991) and that they put relationships at the center and people at the margins (Cherryholmes 1988). Structuralism has also been critiqued for being ahistorical as it focuses on structure at a point in time. Poststructuralism seeks, then, to reinsert the subject into the question of language and the production of meaning, wherein differences operate in a positive manner—not only according to binary oppositions (Pheby 1988).

Most celebrated for his concept of "difference", that which means both to defer and differ, Derrida sought to deconstruct the metaphysical definition of Being as some timeless self-identity or presence to show that difference precedes presence rather than the contrary (Kearney 1984). In that deconstruction, he seeks to undermine the notion that meaning, knowledge, and therefore subjectivity, are stable predictable entities. Difference is designated as that which denies the distinction between or separation of signifier (sign, image) and signified (concept, meaning). In other words, meaning is never immediately present in a sign, since it is always what the sign is not and so is in a way absent from the sign (Martusewicz 1992). In this sense, the subject can never be fully present to itself since, due to the effect of language, it is constantly shifting.

Levinas, likewise, argues that Western philosophy seeks to reduce difference and "otherness" to the category of the "same" (Kearney 1984), and as such it is a totalizing philosophy. Over and against this tradition he proposes an ethics of transcendence based on the primacy of the other over the same; in it he states, the person or the "I does not begin with itself in some pure moment of autonomous self-consciousness but in relation with the other, for whom it remains forever responsible" (Kearney 1984, p. 48). In contrast to Heidegger, Levinas maintains that one's relation to the other is ultimately prior to his ontological relation to self. He puts forward a meontological version of subjectivity (beyond Being); in it I is defined as a subjectivity, as a singular person, as an "I," precisely because of being exposed to the other. As he says, "The other haunts our ontological existence and keeps the psyche awake, in a state of vigilant insomnia" (Kearney 1984, p. 63). This ethics of transcendence is a disruption to our Being-in-the-world which opens us up to the other; the approach to the face is the most basic mode of responsibility.

The vulnerability of the face summons the call to care and begins to disrupt our tension between the technological and the concern about Being that we found at the root of our being called to care. We might give heed now to a different part of that tension—beyond Being. As Levinas says, "The ethical exigency to be responsible for the other undermines the ontological primacy of the meaning of Being; it unsettles the natural and political positions we have taken up in the world and predisposes us to a meaning that is other than Being, that is otherwise than Being" (Kearney 1984, p. 59). If we view our response to the call to care as a response to the claim of the other, we can understand deconstruction as arising from the experience of difference, as it opens up an ethics that experiences the claim not of presence but of absence, not of identity but of difference.

Deconstruction, then, is always responsible with a double gesture, says Caputo (1987), wherein it attends to claims both by responding to them and to see what they have excluded. In doing so, "the old paradigm is made to tremble and a new configuration arises out of its shaking" (1987, p. 218). We must realize, though, as Caputo warns, that every paradigm is a fiction—a way of laying things out. If there is ever to be an understanding more deeply construed, we should not be searching for the latest philosophical standpoint but should seek an element of "movement," which Caputo finds in the Kierkegaardian notion of "repetition":

> Repetition "answers" what is calling to it in what it has been, "responds" to what is possible, makes a rejoinder which consists in bringing forth something for which. . .up to now only has been obscurely groped. The rejoinder. . .is a rebuff. . .of the inertial weight of the past. It is a living response which speaks against, protests, disavows the weight of a tradition which has become leaden and lifeless; effecting the possible is "revolutionary," while clinging to the past is "conservative." There is thus a deconstructive moment in repetition, a moment of countermovement. . .of

rebuttal...which rejects that whose only authority is its prior actuality. Repetition aims at not the actual but the possible. Possibility is higher than actuality. (1987, p. 91)

We want the result of our inquiry, through the responses that we make, to offer up a new way of seeing our practice, effecting an intellectual transformation of the categories themselves. As we begin our response to the call, the categories of inquiry modes or orientations might be considered in the words of Lather (1990) more as provisional constructions rather than as systematic formulations. Through the deconstructive process, we want to radically dislocate the categories and positions that have come to be taken for granted.

The Empirical/Instrumental Response (Control)

The curing approach to health care regards health care as technology, the sense of which is derived from the applied medical science model (Bishop & Scudder 1990). When practice is reduced to applied science or technology, persons are treated as objects; their humanity is denied as they become things determined by natural forces. When applied science replaces practice, practice then degenerates into technique. To learn the techniques of how to give health care in order to cure or heal and to use technological equipment and processes for that end illustrates what Bishop and Scudder call "calculative thinking," wherein we learn how to do something but neglect the meaning of what we are doing. If we consider the language that is used to reflect an instrumental response to care (means to an end), such as *giving* care, learning the skills necessary to use equipment and carrying out procedures, mastering techniques, learning problem solving skills for detecting symptoms, and so forth, our concern is what we *do* with implements/tools and techniques. If we consider instead what the proliferation of technological apparatus and our use of it does to us and those upon whom we use it, we might keep open the instrumental power of technology in a properly human context (Burch 1986). To understand the technological rather than to control it, we would have to develop a new relationship to it. To confront the technological means to confront alienation and what it means to dwell in the world— to truly learn what it means to be at home in the world. So what, then, would be our responsibility here in the call to care? What has been excluded in an instrumental call to care? We might consider that the technics (processes and products of a technological practice) are more significant for what they make possible than for what they are (a Heideggerian notion). For example, when tools or equipment or electronic processes are used, they always open up some aspect of the environment to experience by referring beyond the equipment or tools (Heidegger 1962). We put *ourselves* into these technics and incorporate them as extensions of our experience that lead to other experience—in relation to others with whom we engage in the use of these implements and processes. Our response, then, might be to reflect on the technological phenomenologically and hermeneutically—to describe and be aware of our experience of the technological as coming to question it, rather than seeing it as a problem to be solved (Heidegger, 1977). The response to a problem concerns what we *do*, whereas our response to questions concerns who we *are* as humans. In all questions, it is we ourselves, our having and doing, thinking and being together that is at issue. The technological can be seen as positive in the sense of granting a perspective that allows one to control and order the world. It becomes negative when it opens the world as material for unlimited instrumental action only, where it tends to close off other possibilities for human dwelling and thinking, the caring, mediative, creative aspects of our Being (Burch 1986). Olson (1986) says the nurse must remember that the homeland of the heart gives meaning to technological care.

We might consider what an instrumental response to the call to care excludes in Bergum's (1985) exploration of how the use of a fetal monitor estranges us, disrupts a bond that existed between persons. She raises the question, How does the experience with the fetal monitor affect the woman's relations to those around her, to her unborn child, and even to herself? The contrast between the medical language and the lived language of the mother is stark, to such an extent, Bergum says, that the machine speaks rather than the woman. The woman's face is no longer really seen; instead, the monitor is watched. One woman described the experience as losing a sense of her own contractions, as hearing and experiencing her baby outside herself. The management and control environment of the machine as a caregiving device began to rob her of her own bodily felt sense of birth giving. *What has been excluded by what calls itself care here?* In bypassing the woman's body, does the other become the machine? What changes when we are called by a machine rather than the person? What does this difference give rise to? Might it be that the revealing essence of technology, of which Heidegger speaks, has come into presence here? Through such revealing we recognize the need for a reassessment of what it means to be human, that which has become absent through the presence of the machine. Might it be *choice* that is made possible here? And then does the question become, How do we come to understand that question as we bear our ethical responsibility and divert our gaze back again toward the face of the mother? Might it also be a revealing of how metaphysical thinking re-presents that which is already present, and if we are to overcome this tradition, which relates to people and things and even being as such in this manner, we must move to a thinking that responds and recalls (Levin 1989). We must cease being with people, then, in ways that re-present them as objects. We must recall a bodily felt sense of listening that the fetal monitor sought to re-present in the face of the machine. Two questions, then, might be, How may our hearing be developed so that we can respond appropriately to the call? What, then, might the hermeneutic response offer?

The Hermeneutic/Understanding Response (Being)

The ultimate hermeneutic response is a movement in care—the countermovement to the pull of withdrawal (Caputo 1987). Through a hermeneutic response, we are challenged to ask what we mean by care and what makes it possible for us to speak, think, and act in the ways we do (Smith 1991).

To be human is to be interpretive, for the very nature of the human realm is interpretive. Interpretation is not a tool for knowledge; it is the way human beings are, and experience itself is formed through interpretation of the world. Hermeneutics is the foundational practice of Being itself; in such practice, interpretation is the means by which the nature of Being is disclosed. Interpretation, then, is the primordial condition of human self-understanding.

In Heidegger (1962) we come to a point where hermeneutics is linked with phenomenology. For Heidegger, knowing and understanding are not fundamentally epistemological questions but ontological ones. Knowing and understanding are part of the larger question of what it means to Be. The task of ontology is to explain Being itself. Ontology, then, must become phenomenology as it turns to the process of understanding and interpretation through which things appear as human existence is revealed. All of this, in turn, means that ontology, as phenomenology of Being, becomes a hermeneutics of existence (Hultgren 1989). The mode of Being that is proper to human beings—or the self—is expressed in terms of existence, by which is meant a "standing out toward." This is a way of actually relating to the world that indicates one's intentionality and self-transcendence (reaching beyond self). In response to this fundamental relation, an analysis of human existence must start with Being-in-the-world. True understanding is the result of human engagement in the world.

Derrida's contention is that insofar as Heidegger asks about the essence of truth or the meaning of Being, he still speaks the language of a metaphysics of presence, which looks upon meaning as something preexisting, that is, something to be discovered (Bernstein 1986). But Caputo (1986) suggests that, to Heidegger, hermeneutics means a recovering of origins, a return to the more primordial, which has nothing to do with nostalgia for presence but everything to do with courage for repetition. Repetition has to do not with a past actuality, with a presence lost, but with a presence yet to be realized, with the possible.

If we consider Heidegger's hermeneutics as an attempt at the recovery of meaning, a knowing again, interpretation is the recovery of a prior understanding for which we have heretofore lacked words. Hermeneutics uncovers because it recovers; it brings us to stand in a place we already are. As Caputo (1987) says: "Any exercise in hermeneutical interpretation comes down to its ability to provoke in us the ultimate hermeneutic response: *That* is what we are looking for. That puts into words what we have all along understood about ourselves" (p. 81). In a transformation of the hermeneutic circle from a part-whole relationship to a phenomenological circle of implicit and explicit, prethematic, and thematic, repetition and retrieval restore a mystery, the absence in *Dasein* (Being-in-the-world):

> The call of conscience is a call back to our being thrown Being-in-the-world. The caller of the call of conscience is *Dasein* itself (in its authentic Being), and that which is called is also *Dasein* itself (in its inauthenticity), and what is said to be *Dasein* in the call is to become itself, to be the being that it already is to take up its authentic potentiality for Being. Here there is an existential circle: *Dasein* calls itself to become itself...and the structure of the movement is circular: from *Dasein* to *Dasein*; to become the being that we already are, to be...that which we have all along. (Caputo 1986, p. 429)

What, then, is our responsibility here with respect to the call to care? Might it be the recovery of nursing concerned primarily with care rather than cure as Bishop and Scudder (1990) point to, a recovery wherein nursing practice is viewed as fundamentally moral rather than scientific? We would then be drawn into the significance of relation—how we *are* with one another as we meet each "other" in care. Olson (1986), in trying to understand the life of illness, suggests that care is the *Being* of Being-there in reference to Heidegger's essence of human experience; nurses are the *there* of Being-there. She also illuminates the sense of Heidegger's "*Verfall*"—a falling away from self that is not a genuine Being-with others. Yet this inauthentic way of being generates a longing for something more. Experiencing what is inauthentic allows one to hope for what is authentic. *Dasein* and hope, then, are the reaching forward of care.

If we consider what has been excluded in the original Greek meaning of caring found in *logos* itself, a belonging to each other in community, we can again find a retrieval/revealing in Olson's work with understanding illness. She suggests that the attitude of care is both hidden and revealed in commonly used medical terms such as *cardiology, nephrology,* and *neurology,* the suffix in each of these words being derived from *logos.* Cardiology might mean to speak about care for the heart in a way that listens to, cares for, the meaning of the heart in the life of a human being, in the life of a community. She says that it is *logos* that calls us first, not to an analysis of *what is,* but to an individual *responsiveness* to *what is.* How might we allow the *ology* words to become what they were intended to be, then, in our practice, as we *respond* to the is-ness of care? The good of understanding *is* care.

Hermeneutic inquiry begins with an attempt to understand the question itself—learning to see what needs to be questioned. To Gadamer (1975), the working out of the hermeneutic situation means establishing the right horizon (vantage point) of inquiry, one in which the question is evoked by the encounter with tradition. Since, for Gadamer, it is the nature of a tradition to exist in the medium of language, the integration of interpretation, understanding, and application in relation to the text we seek to understand is an idea central to his philosophic hermeneutics. Language is the medium in which tradition conceals itself and in which it is also transmitted. Experience itself occurs in and through language. It is Gadamer's assertion, then, that human understanding as such is historical, linguistic, and dialectical (Hultgren 1989). The dialectic of question and answer works out a fusion of horizons (range of vision that can be seen from a particular standpoint). In coming to understand with others, we can learn to amend some of our prejudices and come to a richer understanding. He argues, though, that because of our historicity, we cannot fully transcend the prejudices of the tradition to which we belong.

To deconstruct this view would be to question the movement of tradition. Gadamer remains within the tradition that he regards as inescapable, and he seems to project a conservative preservation of what is at work in the tradition. Caputo (1988) suggests that Gadamer is too preoccupied with the fusion of horizons (a digestion of the other), whereas he argues that in deconstruction there is a more radical toleration for a plurality of voices—not bent on assimilating the other but on letting the other be (*Gelassenheit*).

In Gadamer's hermeneutics the other appears as a question, but with Derrida the other appears as a claim. For Gadamer the other is a partner in dialogue in a homogeneous space, whereas the other for Derrida is heard more in a tangled maze of messages, a colloquy. We might, then, suggest what needs to be questioned here with respect to our response to care: What is it about the nursing tradition that has given over nursing as care to the scientific model of nursing as care? How might the original response to care be recovered? What is it about care that has not yet been articulated? What voices might we hear? Will we know when we have arrived at the *logos* (care in community)? What does that meaning and place include/exclude? What might it become? What are the power relations that deconstruction might tend to disrupt? What, then, might be a critical response to care?

Critical/Emancipative Response (Reason)

Relationships of domination exist across a broad spectrum of institutions in society where people have power over other people. The very structures of our social institutions and the predominant norms, values, and beliefs of our society serve to create, sanction, and reinforce such relationships (Kreisberg 1992). The health care system is no exception. As Street (1992) acknowledges:

> The legitimation of medicine is a process by which medicine operates as an institution of social control reproducing the dominant ideology of healthcare in a hegemonic relationship with the state...This hierarchical ordering of knowledge affords superiority to knowledge produced by the natural sciences and used in the practice of medicine and medical technology while denigrating practical knowledge that forms the basis of much of the distinct knowledge of paramedical disciplines and nursing. (p. 30)

At the center of critical theory's response to domination is a reflective critique of socially unnecessary constraints on human freedom (Schroyer 1973), a critique that entails a struggle to break down structures and patterns that dehumanize and disempower. In replacement, it seeks to cultivate forms of relationship that provide affirmation, nurturance, hope, and a sense of possibility. In the context of nursing, such critical scholarship is reflected in patterns of thought and action that challenge institutionalized power relations or relations of domination in the social reality of nursing (Thompson 1987). Some of those realities beginning to be challenged are the accepted superiority of the technical knowledge of doctors, the sexual division of hospital labor, stereotyping of the doctor/nurse/patient roles, devaluation of nurturant knowledge, uniforms as technologies of power, invisibility of patients, constant observation and visibility dialectic of nurses, structured relations to discourage talking and writing about clinical practice, and conflict between oral culture and written culture, to name a few (Street 1992).

Critical social theory enables nurses to examine socially constructed realities, through which meanings of nursing practice and caring are created, and power relations, which shape and form the consciousness of the nurse. It therefore seeks to uncover the social and historical factors that have shaped both the nurse and the clinical setting. Critical social theory assumes people are potentially capable of altering repressive forces that inhibit their development. It views society and knowledge as a human construction that can be altered through human understanding of the taken-for-granted structures that form the fiber of human life in society (Coomer 1989) and focuses on what might be possible in furthering the development of individuals or groups in society. Stimulating a person or group of people to think about such possibilities for change is the aim of Habermas's (1973) critical social theory. The underlying interest of critical theory is emancipation, which is acquired by ideology critique and self-reflection. In the inquiry process, self-reflection is designed to enlighten and build communicative competence and to free persons from technical control; this is the central task of Habermas's critical perspective. His theory of communicative competence is an ethical theory of self-realization that transposes the source of human ideals onto language and discourse, whereby a conception of an ideal form of life in which rational autonomy served by the emancipatory interest can be realized (Carr & Kemmis 1986).

As much as Habermas has contributed to the development of critical theory in the United States, his work does come under criticism, from feminist scholars, particularly, and from those who have sought a postmodern turn to a discourse of plurality, difference, and multi-narratives (Giroux 1991; Lather 1991). Identifying Habermas as the "last" great rationalist, Bernstein (1986) shows Habermas's concern for ground through his communicative action and discourse. Giroux (1991) analyzes Habermas's defense of modernism as an unfinished emancipatory project, particularly the rule of reason. He suggests that modernism frames culture within rigid boundaries that both privilege and exclude around the categories of race, class, gender, and ethnicity and that the discourse becomes an organizing principle for constructing borders reproductive of relations of domination, subordination, and inequality. Postmodernism, on the other hand, is framed within the contexts of shifting identities and the remapping of borders, calling attention to the sphere of culture as a shifting social and historical construction. It has developed a power-sensitive discourse that helps subordinated and excluded groups to make sense of their own social worlds and histories, while offering opportunities to produce new vocabularies by which to shape and define their identities. Lather (1991) also seeks a critical appropriation of postmodernism in the interests of emancipation, turning from dominant power to a focus on oppositional discourses of criticism and resistance. Her interest is in generating "ways of knowing that can take us beyond ourselves" (p. 2).

A critical appropriation of deconstruction would enable nurses to deconstruct the ideological, political, and historical elements of nursing discourse and practice, particularly with respect to caring, as the interest is here in this book. Such discourse would disrupt power relations and create new narratives through which a better social order for nursing, and ultimately caring, might be imagined and struggled for. Abel and Nelson (1990) write about caring as social because it speaks to our survival as a species, rather than as isolated individuals. They define caring as a "species activity that includes everything that we do to maintain, continue and repair our world so that we can live in it as well as possible" (p. 40). They do not assume that women have more of a special ability to do this than men. To speak of caring in those terms allows for the possibility of transforming political discourse around caring and disrupting the binary oppositions of public/private, right/duty, and love/labor. Abel and Nelson call for "caring with autonomy," a way of life that would bring the dichotomies together, a way of life that values caring and negates subservient attitudes.

Street (1992) calls for a similar bringing together of dichotomous oppositions. Her critical ethnography seeks to display how the damaging consequences of adapting to the norms of the oppressor (doctors and hierarchical relations) lead to a marginal status for the oppressed (nurses), whereby the oppressed (nurses) reject their own nurturant characteristics when faced with those valued by the dominant medical model. Drawing upon Foucault's (1980) "power/knowledge" concept, which examines relationships between power and knowledge and the way in which oppressive practices are maintained, accommodated, or resisted within nursing practice, she also recognizes the limitations of that concept, namely the lack of utopian hope and the single-minded focus on domination. Street acknowledges that nurses are not mere passive recipients of oppression, that they are capable of reflecting on the process of their own nursing practice, and that nurturant activities are essential in bringing these practices to light. She therefore seeks a dialectical relationship between power/knowledge and nurturance/knowledge.

What has been excluded by what calls itself "care" from a critical perspective? Without the help of hermeneutics or deconstruction, the nurturant voice called for by persons with concrete needs for care can, through argumentative discourse, be drowned out by the voice of reason and power. Much more is required than a common analysis of oppression; sometimes the very analysis itself becomes oppressive in the hands of those who would designate themselves as the "emancipatory vanguard"—Giroux's (1991, p. 229) name for those who would seek to shape social conditions and history according to their own narratives and thereby become the "omniscient narrators." As much as power relations that are exploitive need to be unmasked, this cannot be done at the expense of losing a language that is hopeful/hope-full or careful/care-full. Discussions of the relationships between power and knowledge in nursing need to take account of the people engaging in those actions. An emancipatory nursing knowledge develops from the experience of engaging in nursing care, experience that is essentially nurturant; Street's (1992) combination of power/knowledge with nurturance/knowledge offers a hopeful discourse dialectic for transformative practice *and* a valuing of the *power of care*. Rather than establishing more rigid border patrols to prevent the crossing of discourse communities, we might instead develop opportunities to meet across boundaries (this the subject of Giroux's 1992 book, *Border Crossings*). One crossing that seems to offer hope for the discourse on care as we struggle to understand what it means to be called to care is that of radical hermeneutics (Caputo 1987), which has moved hermeneutics beyond Being through its deconstructive turn and then back again through the notion of retrieval—a laying out and a fetching back. It provides a kind of thinking that is at once hermeneutic and deconstructive, both unsettling and recuperative, and in its exposure to the flux allows for a deeper understanding of beings that we are and, as is our concern, beings that we are in caring.

A Radical Hermeneutic Response (Beyond Being)

Since Caputo's work is a deconstruction of Heidegger's hermeneutics, begun by Heidegger himself, the problematic it takes up is the metaphysics of being as presence. Caputo's project is to show how hermeneutics in *Being and Time* is already on the way beyond Being as he distinguishes three elements of Being: (1) the Being that is to be understood, (2) the initial determination of its Being (meaning of Being), and (3) that upon which the projecting of Being is carried out (that which gives rise to Being). As Caputo (1987) says: "To think Being is to remain within the first projective cut, but to think the meaning of being is to make a hermeneutic determination of so radical a sort that it leaves metaphysics and its 'Being' behind. When the hermeneutic situation is fully radicalized, we are carried beyond Being to that in which it 'maintains itself,' to that which produces Being as an effect" (p. 85). It is this third interest, then, that Caputo says drew Heidegger into the meaning of what he calls "radical hermeneutics," the willingness to stay in play, to stay with the flux, and that the matter of concern in Heidegger is not Being but "beyond" Being. As much as Heidegger might have been misunderstood or misinterpreted, he was not seeking to propose a grand theory of Being that would lead to the one true meaning of Being. He was not, therefore, even interested in the message or meaning of Being in the traditional sense, but he was interested in the delivery service (that which allows Being to come to pass, *Ereignis*).

Authenticity is directly tied in to this hermeneutic of repetition in which Being and becoming are fused through resisting solid foundations and keeping alive the unrest. As an existential hermeneutic, it wants to recall us to ourselves and to restore our authentic selfhood and Being-with others. As a hermeneutic phenomenology, it seeks to recover an understanding in which we already stand. Recovery is the life of hermeneutics, and deconstruction is but a moment through which it passes. As Caputo says, "there is no hermeneutic recovery without deconstruction and no deconstruction not aimed at recovery" (1987, p. 65). A cautious humility and compassion are the virtues that staying in the play of the flux with the other bring about, the play being characterized by an ethics of dissemination bent on dispersing power clusters. An ethics of dissemination is an ethics of otherness. It is the concern for the other that is at the core of Levinas's ethics of transcendence, which he calls the "interhuman relationship." "The interhuman realm can thus be construed as a part of the disclosure of the world as presence. But it can also be considered from another perspective—the ethical...as a theme of justice and concern for the other as other, as a theme of love and desire which carries us beyond the finite Being of the world as presence" (Kearney 1984, p. 56). It is when I experience the voice of the other that there is a breaking of silence in my world centered on I, a breaking that decenters my universe (van Manen 1991).

Caputo's ethics of dissemination proceeds by way of a great distrust of schemas and foundations; radical hermeneutics causes the ground to give way, exposing the flux at certain breaking points in the habits and practices of our existence. "Something breaks through because the constraints we impose upon things breaks down...What breaks down in the breakthrough is the spell of conceptuality, the illusion that we have somehow or another managed to close our conceptual fists around the nerve of things, that we have grasped the world round about" (Caputo 1987, p. 270). Radical hermeneutics arises, then, at the point of breakdown and loss of meaning. The face and body lend discourse a support as places of opening and breakthrough, the face of suffering being that which puts teeth into the mystery of the other.

What does this mean then in relation to the call to care? As Caputo (1987) says, suffering exposes the vulnerability of human existence by creating an inverted world:

> In the face of suffering the constructs of onto-theo-logic are exposed for what they are, the confidence of common sense is refuted, the acuity of science and the agility of *"phronesis"* are reduced to silence...It is the best "testimony" (we are, after all, outside the realm where arguments and counterarguments settle anything definitely) for the flux which swirls all around us. The look of one whose powers are withering, of a young life being wasted...the familiar structures of our practices and everyday beliefs shatter, breaking down and breaking open. (p. 278)

This is the place where caring is called forward and nurses are constantly in the flux. The struggle with the other in suffering brings one beyond Being. As the following chapters examine the themes of vulnerability, authenticity, and structure, the opposition between technical determination and the desire to "Be" with others in caring offer new possibilities for hearing and seeing the call to care.

References

Abel, E. K., & Nelson, M. K. (1990). *Circles of care: Work and identity in women's lives*. Albany: State University of New York Press.

Aoki, T. T. (1991). *Inspiriting curriculum and pedagogy: Talks to teachers*. Edmonton, Alberta: University of Alberta, Department of Secondary Education.

Atkinson, P., Delamont, S., & Hammersley, M. (1988). Qualitative research traditions: A British response to Jacob. *Review of Educational Research, 58* (2), 231–50.

Bergum, V. K. (1985). *Ear on the belly: A question of fetal monitors* (Occasional Paper No. 38). Edmonton, Alberta: University of Alberta, Department of Secondary Education.

Berman, L. M., Hultgren, F. H., Lee, D., Rivkin, M. S., & Roderick, J. A. (1991). *Toward curriculum for being: Voices of educators.* Albany: State University of New York Press.

Bernstein, R. J. (1986). What is the difference that makes a difference? Gadamer, Habermas, and Rorty. In B. R. Wachterhauser (Ed.), *Hermeneutics and modern philosophy* (pp. 343–76). Albany: State University of New York Press.

Bishop, A. H., & Scudder, J. R., Jr. (1990). *The practical, moral, and personal sense of nursing: A phenomenological philosophy of practice.* Albany: State University of New York Press.

Burch, R. (1986). Confronting technophobia: A topology. *Phenomenology + Pedagogy, 4,* 3–19.

Caputo, J. D. (1986). Hermeneutics as the recovery of man. In B. R. Wachterhauser (Ed.), *Hermeneutics and modern philosophy* (pp. 416–45). Albany: State University of New York Press.

Caputo, J. D. (1987). *Radical hermeneutics: Repetition, deconstruction, and the hermeneutic project.* Bloomington: Indiana University Press.

Caputo, J. D. (1988). Beyond aestheticism: Derrida's responsible anarchy. *Research in Phenomenology, 18,* 59–73.

Carr, W., & Kemmis, S. (1986). *Becoming critical.* Philadelphia: Falmer Press.

Cherryholmes, C. H. (1988). *Power and criticism: Postructural investigations in education.* New York: Teachers College Press.

Coomer, D. L. (1989). Introduction to critical inquiry. In F. H. Hultgren & D. L. Coomer (Eds.), *Alternative modes of inquiry in home economics research* (pp. 167–84). Peoria, IL: Glencoe.

Culler, J. (1991, March). *Fostering post-structuralist thinking.* Paper presented at the annual meeting of the American Educational Research Association, San Francisco.

Foucault, M. (1980). Two lectures. In C. Gordon (Ed.), *Power and knowledge: Selected interviews and other writings by Michel Foucault, 1972–1977.* New York: Pantheon.

Gadamer, H-G. (1975). *Truth and method.* New York: Crossroad.

Giroux, H. A. (Ed.) (1991). *Postmodernism, feminism, and cultural politics: Redrawing educational boundaries.* Albany: State University of New York Press.

Giroux, H. A. (1992). *Border crossings.* New York: Routledge.

Habermas, J. (1973). *Theory and practice* (J. Viertel, Trans.). Boston: Beacon Press.

Heidegger, M. (1962). *Being and time* (J. Macquarrie & E. Robinson, Trans.). New York: Crossroad. (Original work published 1927)

Heidegger, M. (1977). *The question concerning technology and other essays* (W. Lovitt, Trans.). New York: Harper & Row.

Huebner, D. (1987). The vocation of teaching. In F. S. Bolin & J. M. Falk (Eds.), *Teacher renewal: Professional issues, personal choices* (pp. 17–29). New York: Teachers College Press.

Hultgren, F. H. (1989). Introduction to interpretive inquiry. In F. H. Hultgren & D. L. Coomer (Eds.), *Alternative modes of inquiry in home economics research* (pp. 37–59). Peoria, IL: Glencoe.

Kearney, R. (1984). *Dialogues with contemporary continental thinkers: The phenomenological heritage.* Dover, NH: Manchester University Press.

Kreisberg, S. (1992). *Transforming power: Domination, empowerment, and education.* Albany: State University of New York Press.

Lashley, M. (1990, October). *Experiencing the call to care: Creating authentic structures for responsible caregiving.* Paper presented at the Conference on Curriculum Theory and Classroom Practice, Dayton, OH.

Lather, P. (1990, October). *My body, my text: Counter practices of authority in discourses of liberatory education.* Paper presented at the Conference on Curriculum Theory and Classroom Practice, Dayton , OH.

Lather, P. (1991). *Getting smart: Feminist research and pedagogy with/in the postmodern.* New York: Routledge.

Levin, D. M. (1989). *The listening self: Personal growth, social change and the closure of metaphysics.* New York: Routledge.

Levi-Strauss, C. (1972). *Structural anthropology.* Hanmondsworth: Penguin.

Lyotard, J. F. (1989). *The postmodern condition: A report on knowledge.* Minneapolis: University of Minnesota Press.

Margolis, J. (1985). Deconstruction; or, The mystery of the mystery of the text. In H. J. Silverman & D. Ihde (Eds.), *Hermeneutics & deconstruction* (pp. 138–51). Albany: State University of New York Press.

Martusewicz, R. A. (1992). Mapping the terrain of the post-modern subject. In W. F. Pinar & W. M. Reynolds (Eds.), *Understanding curriculum as phenomenological and deconstructed text* (pp. 131–58). New York: Teachers College Press.

Neal, M. (1987). Class drafts for EDIT 788P. University of Maryland.

Olson, C. T. (1986). *How can we understand the life of illness?* Unpublished doctoral dissertation, University of Alberta, Edmonton.

Pheby, K. C. (1988). *Interventions: Displacing the metaphysical subject.* Institute for Advanced Cultural Studies: Maisonneuve Press.

Pinar, W. F., & Reynolds, W. M. (1992). Curriculum as text. In W. F. Pinar & W. M. Reynolds (Eds.), *Understanding curriculum as phenomenological and deconstructed text* (pp. 1–14). New York: Teachers College Press.

Schroyer, T. (1973). *The critique of domination: The origins and development of critical theory.* New York: Braziller.

Slunt, E. (1987). Class drafts for EDIT 788P. University of Maryland.

Slunt, E. T. (1989). Becoming competent: A phenomenological inquiry into its meaning by nursing students. Doctoral dissertation. University of Maryland, College Park. *Dissertation Abstracts International, 51,* 1196B.

Smith, D. (1991). Hermeneutic inquiry: The hermeneutic imagination and the pedagogic text. In E. C. Short (Ed.), *Forms of curriculum inquiry* (pp. 187–209). Albany: State University of New York Press.

Street, A. F. (1992). *Inside nursing: A critical ethnography of clinical nursing practice.* Albany: State University of New York Press.

Thompson, J. L. (1987). Critical scholarship: The critique of domination in nursing. *Advanced Nursing Science, 10*(1), 27–38.

van Manen, M. (1991). *The tact of teaching.* Albany: State University of New York Press.

II

Living the Call as Inquiring Learners

In living the call to care, we found that three major themes became apparent as learners and educators explored together the meaning of expressing one's Being and the meaning of creating curricula and deeper understandings. The themes of vulnerability, authenticity, and structure were found in our research of nursing education. These themes were developed through further interpretative and deconstructive analysis of the texts created from our original research.[1]

Following a call to care inevitably leads to encounters of uncertainty and vulnerability. In chapter 3, Mary explores the tensions and contradictions associated with vulnerability. She describes in an ontological sense new discoveries and deeper understandings that become possible as persons question the meaning of an anxious state of Being.

Emily explores the meaning of authenticity in chapter 4. Readers are asked to reflect upon what happens to the authentic voice of the nurse and the sense of fulfillment in answering a call to care. They are invited to reflect upon and also ponder what it is like to experience the "Being-there," the realness of a genuine relationship with another person.

In chapter 5, Maggie writes about structure and conformity inherent in nursing education curricular practices. The tension and contradictions surrounding these issues may prevent one from nurturing or sustaining a call to care. Questions are proposed that can help us consider possiblities for finding an openness within structure, a direction that is more attuned to persons called to care.

Readers may resonate with the themes of vulnerability, authenticity, and structure and make connections between their own stories and the questions raised in the text. Readers are also invited to join the authors in raising additional questions through dialogue and reflection.

As students, educators, and caregivers we have the potential to be inquiring learners. Therefore we have the potential to open up new possibilities for thinking about nursing and education and for helping persons come to a clearer understanding of what it means to be called to care.

Notes

1. The original texts include the following doctoral dissertations: M. E. Lashley (1989) *Being with the Elderly in Community Health Nursing: Exploring Lived Experience through Reflective Dialogue* Doctoral disseration, University of Maryland, College Park, *Dissertation Abstracts International, 51,* 729A. M. T. Neal (1989) *A Room with a View; Uncovering the Essence of Student Experience in a Clinical Nursing Setting* Doctoral dissertation, University of Maryland, College Park, *Dissertation Abstracts International, 50,* 2847B. E. T. Slunt (1989) *Becoming Competent; A Phenomenological Inquiry into Its Meaning by Nursing Students* Doctoral dissertation, University of Maryland, College Park, *Dissertation Abstracts International, 51,* 1196B.

3

Vulnerability: The Call to Woundedness

Mary Ellen Lashley

As doctoral students interested in alternative approaches to nursing inquiry, my colleagues and I were brought together through our dissertation experiences. Despite varied professional interests and research contexts, we were intrigued to find similar patterns emerging in our works. We found the theme of vulnerability to be particularly prominent in our writings and conversations with students and with one another. Specifically, the theme emerged for each of us in our doctoral studies as we found ourselves moving away from the abstractions of representational thinking and scientific theorizing toward the concreteness of actual experience.

At the completion of our studies, Louise our dissertation advisor, our mentor, colleague, and colaborer in this present text, invited us into her home for an informal conversation about our doctoral education. Through our dialogue, I became more acutely aware of the prominence of the theme of vulnerability, not only in my research, but also in my life. I found a pattern of woundedness within human experience and a compelling desire to understand and to respond more sensitively to persons who encounter wounding experiences.

This section of text represents a weaving of my own personal voice with the voices of Maggie and Emily as we explore together the theme of vulnerability and attempt to come to a clearer understanding of what it means to be touched by human tenderness (George 1990).

Vulnerability: Becoming a Constant Companion to Pain

In a recent public documentary on nursing, a nurse who was interviewed reflected that pain is the constant companion of a good nurse. By being open to experiencing another's pain, one is rendered vulnerable; that is, more prone to injury. Joyce Travelbee (1966), noted nurse theorist and author, sees the crisis of personal vulnerability as an inevitable consequence of the call to care: "No human being can be repeatedly exposed to illness, suffering, and death, without being changed as a result of these encounters. So too the nurse is changed because, in being confronted with the vulnerability of others, she comes face to face with the compelling force of her own vulnerability in a way that cannot be disregarded" (p. 45). The word *vulnerable* stems from the Latin word *vulnus*, meaning "wound" (Skeat 1882). Vulnerability carries with it the notion of being wounded or becoming more prone to injury. As a nurse educator, I find that my students seem to struggle to find meaning in the midst of wounding experiences. Confronted with the realities of suffering, I sense with them the helplessness and vulnerability to isolation, illness, and loss and the fear of one's own destiny that comes in caring for persons experiencing threats to their physical, emotional, and spiritual well-being.

In the following section, the theme of vulnerability is examined for its potential in opening up new possibilities for experiencing the call to care. Questions are also posed to invite further dialogue and reflection. The meaning of vulnerability surfaces through the tensions and contradictions inherent in the development of a professional identity. The ontological risks associated with being rendered vulnerable are seen as inseparable from the call to care. Finally, personal responses to the challenges of vulnerability are explored.

Vulnerability and Professional Identity

The development of a professional identity is an ongoing process filled with tensions and contradictions. In aspiring to develop a sense of competence as part of one's professional identity, one inevitably encounters vulnerability. Vulnerability is experienced as the self is faced with uncertainty.

In the realm of epistemological knowing, the scope of nursing knowledge and the mystery of certain bodily functions is such that an element of the unknown is always present. An inner awareness that competence is still a goal to be achieved and never an end in itself leaves both student and teacher feeling vulnerable.

When the self faces uncertainty, it is often left feeling exposed and unprotected. For example, the epistemological knowing associated with becoming competent as a nurse can be overwhelming for a novice. The process of integrating knowing into being is one that evolves over time. Failure to meet one's own or another's expectations may leave one feeling inadequate and vulnerable. Barriers in relationships are created to protect the self from uncertainty.

In the following passage, a student recounts her experience of assisting a patient when he gave himself an insulin injection:

That was hard for me because I really didn't understand what he was doing clearly. I was afraid he would ask me a question, and I didn't know what I could tell him. It makes me feel so insecure and afraid that someone will ask me something and I won't know the answer and they'll think well, what's she doing here if she doesn't know the answer right away. (Slunt 1989, pp. 125-26)

In this example, the student perceives competence and expert knowing as a source of legitimation for her presence. Justification for Being-there is related to "know[ing] the answer right away" and being able to communicate it efficiently.

Tensions and contradictions also emerge when the self as teacher faces uncertainty. Self-discovery and the possibilities one faces in redefining who one is and what one stands for create many tensions. One cannot remove boundaries or change perspectives without becoming vulnerable. Paradoxically, the vulnerability that comes from self-exposure and opening oneself up to experience tensions and contradictions may restore a sense of direction and create a new awareness of one's situatedness and orientation to the world.

Vulnerability as Inseparable from the Call to Care

As Travelbee (1966) reflects, vulnerability is an inevitable consequence of the call to care. To acknowledge the call to care is to become aware of one's journey into selfhood, to bring into question one's traditions and previous understandings, to openly respond to others, to become comfortable with doubt and uncertainty, and to acknowledge the inevitable risk that comes when one is invited to rethink the personal values and meanings associated with being a teacher, nurse, or person. Such openness and doubt is not due to incompetence but is a manifestation of a life still evolving and a story yet to be told (Huebner 1987).

Rather than approaching the pain of vulnerability as something to be avoided at all costs, it is important to recognize that when one makes a commitment to care for others, one is committing to a relationship that renders one vulnerable and open to experiencing pain. My colleagues and I discovered, in our research, that many persons actually enter nursing because of an experience with personal injury

or because an illness of a family member results in a hospitalization
where they experience ongoing contact with nurses during periods of
"vulnerability," "helplessness," or "total dependency." Here is an example.

> Nursing was not my first choice. My first choice was
> computer programming. At the age of eighteen, when I was a first
> year college student, I was involved in a serious accident, which
> changed my life forever. . .This accident resulted in many serious
> injuries to me and the death of my best friend. Due to my injuries
> I was totally dependent on the nursing staff. It was during this
> hospitalization that my interest in nursing began. (Neal 1990, p. 4)

Frankl (1963) contends that the meaning of one's existence is
discovered through suffering. To live is to suffer. Yancey (1984) observes
that one learns as a servant "at the feet of teachers in the school of
suffering" (p. 91). Indeed, persons are changed by their wounding
experiences. Should one's focus, then, as a professional caregiver, be
on creating healing milieus in the midst of wounding experiences that
assist persons to find meaning in suffering?

Frankl (1963) found, through his concentration camp experiences
during World War II, that to survive, one must find meaning in
suffering. This "will to meaning" is a continual process of striving to
find meaning in one's existence. Travelbee (1966) proposes that a major
purpose of nursing is to assist individuals or families to find meaning
in the experience of illness or suffering. Here, meaning is defined as
the reasons given for life experiences or the "why" of life.

Vulnerability: An Ontological Risk

Such striving for meaning is not without risk, however. Dr. Richard
C. Halverson, Chaplain of the United States Senate, has observed that
some persons relate like marbles: "The fear of vulnerability hardens
them. They protect themselves, allowing no one to penetrate. Being
vulnerable is high risk and they want low risk" (Halverson 1986, p. 67).

It seems as though the nature of this risk is ontological, as its
essential concern is the very Being of persons. This ontological risk
involves facing the joy and the pain of revealing one's innermost, secret
self. Vulnerability involves self-disclosure. To disclose means to unveil,
to make manifest, and to show. In self-disclosure, one makes oneself
known in a different way to oneself and to others. Authentic self-
disclosure requires the courage to be in the midst of threats to Being
(Tillich 1952).

The following excerpt from a student journal reveals the struggle to become and remain open and vulnerable. Her use of language also hints at something about the structure of relatedness in caring encounters.

> I need to extend myself—my secret self to friends—open the windows. Walls need to come down and let the sun shine in. Sometimes I feel so afraid—afraid I'll be left alone. I've been hurt so many times before. I'm tired of trying—still holding back—want to let go completely. (Neal 1989, p. 166)

Vulnerability also surfaces as persons strive to give some attention to their own sense of being. For example, one student wrote:

> I've just got to stop. Stop the music, Stop the talking, stop the racing thoughts—just stop. Face it Nina—Face the pain of growing up. Feel what it's like to be scared, to be alone, to be. Stop running. Stop filling the space with doing. Sit still. Cry. Let it all out. Let it go, only after you face it. You've rationalized, you've gone to others, you've belittled it all, now, now, just let it be.
>
> Not for Maggie, and school, not for reaching Christine (her sister). Not for record's sake—For you. I do know that I have to write and yet I have not. Instead of sitting still—I run around doing. (Neal 1989, p. 179)

The ontological risk associated with self-disclosure may come about when one recognizes one's fundamental relatedness to others. This feeling of relatedness or sense of common humanity may bring one to the realization that the condition of being wounded and finite is universal. Through one's own experience of pain, one may become less rigid, more understanding, and more accepting of another's pain (Blomquist 1989).

Paradoxically, since persons often experience their wounds in an intensely personal way, they may also feel alone and alienated from others. Events and situations that lie beyond human understanding add to this awareness of personal vulnerability. Persons are rendered vulnerable as they experience the jolting of the familiar and expected. Encountering newness and uncertainty is threatening. The potential for harm becomes a feared possibility.

Nursing students express difficulty in seeing patients suffer and in being the ones who may be responsible for inflicting pain. Deep anxiety, guilt, and the fear of failure to preserve life may also weigh heavily on those who feel called to care. Being with others in experiences of illness, suffering, and death necessitates coming face to face with one's own mortality. Helping students to see the relationships between themselves and those who are entrusted to their care brings forth feelings of identification. Recognizing that Being is finite, persons may experience anxiety and despair. This type of anxiety, however, may allow persons to cherish their own Being and to care more deeply about the Being of others (Tillich 1973).

Since the experience of vulnerability carries with it certain inherent risks, indifference, detachment, and denial may emerge as protective responses to guard against distress. Still, being rendered vulnerable may also deepen the nurse's understanding of the human condition and may serve as a common bond uniting him or her with humanity (Travelbee 1966).

The aloneness experienced by caregivers is experiential as well as ontological. Students may experience feelings of being lost when they first step foot in the clinical agency and attempt to adapt to a new environment fraught with ambiguity, uncertainty, and risk. Students may also come to feel lost and abandoned cognitively when they are left alone to make decisions and think things through. Faculty, in making leaps in clinical judgements, may leave the student faltering behind. At times, students may be unable to keep pace with the conceptual leaps made by more experienced practitioners.

Ironically, by becoming an inquirer into one's own presence in teaching, the experienced educator and practitioner also becomes a student, studying and learning about his or her own practice. This type of self-reflection can leave one feeling isolated and lonely. As teacher-researchers, one is rendered vulnerable as one becomes more consciously aware of the meaning of one's experiences and of the stories that are being told and lived out together. One may come to feel very much alone in one's own personal reflections and disclosures.

In my own experience, I question whether I should disclose the vulnerabilities I experience with my students. If so, how much should be disclosed? What type of feelings and experiences should be disclosed? At what point do my self disclosures become more personally therapeutic than educationally sound? On the other hand, when experiences are structured that do not attend to questions of Being, I find that students often express concern over the loss of sense of self that is felt in being consumed in one's role. Persons may experience feelings of powerlessness and meaninglessness if they do not have a strong sense of self-identity, self-worth, and integrity.

The discomfort and the risk that comes in rendering oneself vulnerable may lead one to question whether it is worth the pain. George (1990) reminds us that risking vulnerability to achieve genuine relationships with self and others is worth the risk: "We will not go through life unbitten. But if we don't take the necessary risks, we can go through life untouched by human tenderness" (p. 177).

Responding to the Call of Vulnerability

How do we respond to the call of vulnerability? In what ways do persons respond in the face of ontological risks (risks to Being)? What obstacles must be faced to allow oneself to become vulnerable? What would a nursing curriculum look like that allowed persons to be touched by human tenderness?

Giving priority to 'Being' in a cognitively oriented curriculum is not without risk. Such a confrontation of the difference between knowing about and being with another leads to intimate questioning of oneself as teacher and researcher as one tries to reshape one's understanding and ground practice in the realities of "being" a teacher, articulating that which is unique about the daily life of nursing education. Both joy and pain are experienced as persons seek to renew meaning in their work, to create a meaningful direction, and to resolve to align one's work more closely with one's belief about the inherent worth and dignity of the human person. Rather than being viewed as an expert who imparts knowledge, the emphasis shifts to the inquiry process itself. Such a shift requires that one be open to being influenced as much as one is open to influencing others.

The metaphors used in personal communications with educators and in the literature to describe the response to vulnerability often center around confinement, protection, imprisonment, and the creation of barriers. For example, George (1990) describes her personal experience with vulnerability and isolation as one of breaking out of confinement. Feeling as though she were a prisoner in a cell, she notes that, as she allowed herself to experience genuine, open relationships with others, the cement that held her cell together began to crack. She could see larger beams of light peeping through the cracks and crevices of her cell: "The lights are beginning to warm the soul inside. The cell that for so many years has been hidden, cold, and lonely. Little by little I am spending more time outside my crumbling prison than inside. And life has taken on a whole new meaning" (George 1990, p. 30).

Carson (1990) and Huebner (1987) describe the protective armor a teacher may use to control the flux of uncertainty and the newness inherent within teaching-learning experiences. As teachers, nurses, and caregivers, we often "arm" ourselves for protection from hurt, anxiety, and guilt. Such armor may take the form of explicit objectives, efficiency, a heavy task orientation, and specific rules for communicating with others to promote control and predictability. Such an approach can, at times, foster self-estrangement and diminish the inherent worth and dignity of the person.

The tendency to arm oneself and to guard against injury is not without reason. Many legitimate fears restrict openness and encourage the donning of protective armor. The fear of being exploited, of surrendering control, of being unpleasantly confronted by unresolved conflicts with oneself or others, and the fear of rejection and loss of self-respect discourage disclosure (Conway 1984). Yet openness to the other means entering into the places of nakedness where the armor wears thin. Such a stand requires that one first accept and come to grips with one's own vulnerability (Carson 1990).

According to Carson (1990), "teaching means to live in the flux of the newness of the world and in the play of competence and vulnerability" (p. 14). The use of protective armor may negate the importance of this flux of newness and deny its essential expression. Protective armor should not be used to keep the unexpected to a minimum or to control the more creative and spontaneous engagement of students in their professional worlds (Carson 1990). Persons should not attempt to find ways to completely avoid or overcome vulnerability but rather search for ways to experience vulnerability without being immobilized by it. Allowing vulnerability to be an integral part of teaching, learning, and nursing requires a social context of acceptance and support and a community of individuals able to share risks and to nurture one another's personal stories to disclosure (Huebner 1987).

Several questions surface in light of the dilemmas posed by rendering oneself vulnerable. How may teachers and practitioners be more fully present to students and patients during experiences of vulnerability? What would be essential for allowing vulnerability to unfold in a safe manner? How may one lay claim to a language that is essential to creating a caring pedagogic presence as one encounters vulnerability? Can we acquire the confidence it takes to drop our hesitations and speak more directly about loving our students and those entrusted to our care? May healing milieus be created in the midst of wounding experiences that nurture self-disclosure and openness? Could such milieus be nurturing a new language, a lived language of vulnerability?

A common theme I see in the work of my colleagues is the use of language not traditionally associated with a pedagogic dialogue grounded in a behaviorist orientation. Nursing, like education, has tended to emphasize the language of the behavioral sciences over alternative modes of discourse such as those grounded in theology or philosophy (Bolin 1987). Perhaps, the expression of vulnerability is nurtured through a different kind of discourse, one that addresses ontological issues; that is, a more spiritual discourse.

Such a discourse may allow one to speak more clearly and more freely about the ontological risks surrounding the condition of vulnerability. Such a discourse may also allow one to speak more directly to the notion of *love*. A discourse grounded in vulnerability may help persons to recognize the value of devotion as an act of commitment both to the other and to an unknown future (Mayeroff 1971).

Such a discourse could allow one to speak more directly about the notion of *humility* as a way of overcoming arrogance and self-aggrandizement and recognizing that one's accomplishments are based in part on conditions over which one has no control (Mayeroff 1971). Blomquist (1989) equates humility with authenticity when she writes that humility is "walking in the truth of who you are" (p. 10). Humility may allow one to acknowledge another's perception of oneself, to embrace one's strengths and weaknesses, and to envision forgiveness as a continual process and not a one-time act (Blomquist 1989).

The expression of vulnerability may also bring about *hope* that the person one cares for will grow through one's act of caring and that the present holds many possibilities for shaping the future. Such hope may give one the *courage* needed to take risks and to stand beside another in conditions of ambiguity and uncertainty (Mayeroff 1971).

The discourse associated with the experience of vulnerability may indeed help to create safer, more comforting environments that permit greater tolerance and acceptance of ambiguity and uncertainty. Such a discourse, however, is not without price: "The words I love you involve a price. To love someone as commitment, not as mere feeling, involves a letting go of something. A letting go of oneself. There hangs a price tag to that kind of love. It costs us something of ourselves, that tender, vulnerable self. It opens up to another being and allows us to see us as we are, not what we pretend to be" (George 1990, p. 154).

Could a language that expresses such values ultimately cultivate a more reverential attitude towards persons or, as Peterson (1984) notes, an attitude of awe? Such an attitude would be in keeping with most nursing philosophies, which espouse the importance of respecting the inherent worth and dignity of persons. Could such a language assist one to view all persons as vulnerable, preserved up to the present moment in a world of hurtling automobiles, ravaging diseases, and limitless perils (Peterson 1984)? Could such a language assist persons in recognizing that every meeting with another is a privilege and an awesome experience, full of potential and possibility (Peterson 1984)? Such an awareness may lead one to marvel, to be in awe, and to appreciate more fully the inherent worth and dignity of others.

In following the call to care, one will inevitably encounter vulnerability. This condition of being wounded or more prone to injury is experienced when the self faces uncertainty. The feeling of exposure, loss of protection, and tension and contradiction are inherent in the experience of vulnerability. Vulnerability involves risk taking. These risks are inherently ontological, as persons come to experience the self-alienation, redefinition, and discovery that comes when they are faced with events that lie beyond human understanding. Responses to vulnerability involve a dynamic flux between arming oneself and entering into places of nakedness. Disclosure of the tensions inherent in this flux are illuminated in the context of a spiritual discourse, which may allow one to speak more directly to the personal meanings of vulnerability for oneself and others and to respond to the call to care in the midst of an environment fraught with ambiguity and uncertainty.

References

Blomquist, J. (1989). Of seeds and suffering: Growing spiritually through a divorce. *Weavings: A journal of the Christian spiritual life, IV* (3), 10.

Bolin, F. (1987). Reassessment and renewal in teaching. In F. S. Bolin & J. M. Falk (Eds.), *Teacher renewal: Professional issues, personal choices* (pp. 6–16). New York: Teachers College Press.

Bolin, F. S., & Falk, J. M. (Eds.). (1987). *Teacher renewal: Professional issues, personal choices*. New York: Teachers College Press.

Carson, T. (1990, October). *Pedagogical reflections on reflective practice in teacher education*. Paper presented at the Bergamo Conference on Curriculum Theory and Classroom Practice, Dayton, OH.

Conway, J. (1989). *Friendship*. Grand Rapids: Zandervan Publishers.

Frankl, V. E. (1963). *Man's search for meaning:* (Original work published in 1946) New York: Washington Square Press.

George, D. (1990). *Becoming tender in a tough world*. Nashville: Broadman's Press.

Halverson, R. (1986). *No greater power.* Portland: Multnomah Press.

Huebner, D. (1987). The vocation of teaching. In F. S. Bolin & J. M. Falk (Eds.), *Teacher renewal: Professional issues, personal choices* (pp. 17–29). New York: Teachers College Press.

Mayeroff, M. (1971). *On caring.* New York: Harper & Row.

Neal, M. T. (1989). A room with a view: Uncovering the essence of the student experience in a clinical nursing setting (Doctoral dissertation, University of Maryland, College Park). *Dissertation Abstracts International, 50,* 2847B.

Neal, M. T. (1990, October). *Coming home to our living rooms.* Paper presented at the Bergamo Conference on Curriculum Theory and Classroom Practice, Dayton, OH.

Peterson, E. (1984). Practicing and malpracticing the presence of God. *Leadership,* Fall, pp. 94–99.

Simonson, H. & Magee, J. (Eds.). *Dimensions of Man.* New York: Harper and Row.

Skeat, W. (1882). *An etymological dictionary of the English language.* Oxford: Clarendon Press.

Slunt, E. T. (1989). Becoming competent: A phenomenological inquiry into its meaning by nursing students. (Doctoral dissertation. University of Maryland, College Park). *Dissertation Abstracts International, 51,* 1196B.

Tillich, P. (1952). *The courage to be.* New Haven: Yale University Press.

Tillich, P. (1973). The three types of anxiety and the nature of man. In H. Simonson & J. Magee (Eds.), *Dimensions of man* (pp. 15–18). New York: Harper & Row.

Travelbee, J. (1966). *Interpersonal aspects of nursing.* Philadelphia: F. A. Davis.

Yancey, P. (1984). Helping those in pain, *Leadership,* Spring, pp. 90–97.

4

Living the Call Authentically

Emily Todd Slunt

In researching the meaning of becoming competent for nursing students, I questioned the balance between science and art and between knowing and caring in a nursing education curriculum. The curriculum seems to reinforce a mechanistic, impersonal way of knowing that is focused on the measurement of concrete and specific behaviors. An emphasis on the technical seems to imply a deemphasis on the art or humanistic and caring aspects of nursing.

In reflecting upon my own personal experiences, however, it is the exemplars of caring and compassion that provide the greatest sense of meaning and empowerment. Caring and connecting with others, being authentic, is so much more powerful than the technical, structured activities associated with being a nurse. I wondered what happens to the authentic voice of the student when confronted with the tensions of "performance" in the clinical setting. What happens to the sense of person? I wondered what it is like for a student to experience the Being-there, the realness of a genuine relationship with another person?

The theme of authenticity emerged in our dissertation research as we interpreted and reflected upon text derived from the lived experiences of nursing students. It was a common theme, despite varied research contexts. In our discussions we came to understand authenticity as an issue in nursing today. Much of health care is delivered in impersonal high tech environments with a business-oriented approach to establishing priorities and making decisions. A concern for the authentic voice in living the call to care provides the focus for this chapter.

I explore the meaning of authenticity around the theme of time. The past affects our ability to live the call authentically. Experiences illuminate the meaning of being real or genuine to self and others and provide the grounding for authentic encounters and ways of Being. Questions are raised and the reader is asked to join in dialogue and reflection to produce new levels of understanding and to find new meaning through creation of an inquiring presence. Curriculum recommendations seek to restore a sense of the person being called to care.

Finding a Historical Consciousness

The notion of a historical consciousness means understanding how one's past shapes one's present and future choices and actions. Coming to terms with one's past is accepting responsibility for one's existence. Relph (1976) views authenticity as a complete awareness and acceptance of responsibility for one's existence. Persons are authentic when they acknowledge their freedom to choose, their ability to project a new world of possibility, and their responsibility for self and others (Ricoeur 1981).

Being authentic allows time for reflection and renewal. Reflection is used to break the spell of naivete by calling into question self-responsibility and ability to respond to others. It involves confronting one's own motivations and alternatives (Paterson & Zderad 1976). For Caputo (1987) it is a continual search and quest, a movement: "Authenticity means unrest, disquiet, uneasiness, agitation, keeping off balance, resisting the illusion of stability and solid foundations" (p. 200).

Human beings come with their own unique histories and bring their own stories. Through stories persons can listen to the past in a way that enables new meaning to become apparent. Mandy, a student, reflected upon her experience with patient suffering:

> There's days that I go home and I can't stop thinking about certain things that may have happened or wonder how a patient feels now and how anxious they must be now because of the situation and the pain that they're feeling. It does bother me. It always has, I think. I remember as a younger person having to visit people in the hospital. I remember being very uncomfortable and feeling I had to leave and go to the bathroom or go outside and get fresh air because it was overwhelming. And I don't feel that any more or I wouldn't be here, but I think it just is a feeling that I have sometimes. (Slunt 1989, p. 119)

The story reveals contradictions and unearths questions. The caring continues at home. The student hurts knowing that the patient is hurting. Through disclosure, Mandy caught a glimpse of her own history and the meaning persons in need have had to her. In revisiting her discomfort with suffering, Mandy affirms her own strength while also catching a glimpse of the anxiety and care at her inner core.

Being authentic means feeling more centered, more whole, more creative, and more free. Greene (1973) defines authenticity as the "sense of the person one ought to be" (p. 286). It means a "homecoming"—a hermeneutic experience that returns self to a dwelling place, a dwelling place that reinitiates nature. Hermeneutics returns us to ourselves, brings us home (Caputo 1987). We are allowed to be who we are, to accept limitation and go forth. Making explicit the thematic claims of the past is the way we gain insight and escape from them.

With a heightened awareness of oneself and others, one reflects upon beliefs and relationships with others. It is self in relationship with others that allows the authentic self to be understood and affirmed. We know the meaning of an event when we come face to face with another. Something passes from one to the other as persons are seen as being in need (Levinas 1987). The self is transformed as we come to know our world and to know self (Morgan 1983).

Living Authentically in the Present

The term *authenticity*, derived from the Greek word *authentikos* encompasses the notion of being real or genuine. "Authenticity means being oneself, honestly, in one's relations with his fellows. It means taking the first step at dropping pretense, defenses, and duplicity" (Jourard 1971, p. 133).

Authenticity also means living the call into nursing or teaching. An inner summons moves one in a particular direction; a calling liberates that which is possible. A calling is discovered. Persons ask, "What must I do?" If a person can recognize the essence of the call, it may be possible to recognize the power within self that brought that call into action. Van Manen (1984) postulates that in the calling one may find Being. According to Paul Tillich, "The power of the self is its self-centeredness" or self-awareness (Tillich 1954, p. 52). An empowered person is more acceptable to self, and personal strength or comfort with one's own Being is the foundation for reaching out to the other, for living the call into nursing. The call comes from Being and opens possibilities for encounters with others, encounters that are more authentic and meaningful: "Finding the call to care means knowing the other as well as self. To care for someone, I must know many things. I must know, for example who the other is, what his powers and limitations are, what his needs are, and what is conducive to his growth; I must know how to respond to his needs and what my own powers and limitations are" (Mayeroff 1971, p. 13).

It is through the power of caring that a nurse or teacher may fulfill the "call to care." Heidegger (1962) believes that care motivates persons to make the choices that would realize possibilities and potential and that Being or self is expressed through care. The calling of self to itself summons a return from lostness and reflects concern for others (Heidegger 1962). The care that constitutes one's Being, therefore, includes awareness and care for self and helping others reach towards possibilities and potential.

Heidegger (1962) describes two ways of caring. "Leaping in," and dominating or "leaping ahead," and liberating while considering the other's potentiality of Being. "Leaping ahead" or "leaping forth" is Heidegger's authentic mode; he states the "it helps the other to become transparent to himself in his care and to become free for it" (p. 159). Scudder (1990) expands upon Heidegger's description. It is the "leaping ahead" or authentic care wherein the other is helped to care for one's own Being.

Caring relationships illuminate a sense of trust, and Being is realized through care. However, as Patricia Benner notes: "The power of caring is underestimated and undervalued in this era when status, mastery, control, and knowledge...are seen as the sources of power...To abandon the power inherent in caring relationships is to sell out but, worse yet, it is to become alienated from our own identity and to thwart our own excellence" (Benner 1984, p. 216).

Authenticity is expressed through care and knowing in an interpersonal sense. An authentic nurse would provide care creatively in response to particular patient needs (Scudder 1990). During moments of genuine presence, in reaching and touching another person, one finds power in self, as being autonomous, good, worthwhile, and responsible. Nurses are challenged to develop the use of self as a basis of nursing care (Watson 1981). In using power found within oneself, the nurse is often able to reach beyond the surface of physical symptoms or behavioral manifestations. An authentic presence is of sufficient power to penetrate an outer armor of objectivity and its associated repelling force. An elusive inner self is more likely to be discovered through connecting with another's genuine presence.

The nurse in the therapeutic use of self rejects approaching the patient-client as an object and strives instead to actualize an authentic personal relationship between two persons. The individual is considered as an integrated, open system incorporating movement toward growth and fulfillment of human potential. An authentic personal relation requires the acceptance of others in their freedom to create themselves and the recognition that each person is not a fixed entity, but constantly engaged in the process of becoming. (Jourard 1971, p. 19)

Nurses and educators are privileged to have the ongoing, daily opportunity to affect the lives of others. In working with both patients and students, we are in close physical proximity to making a difference. In coming face to face we take the first step towards creating an enduring interpersonal bond, one that is capable of withstanding physical separation. An enduring bond is sustained through an authentic relationship and supports the potential and growth of other in the "process of becoming." In conceptualizing personal meanings we are able to sustain connection and an authentic presence even when persons are not physically present to one another.

"Nursing is an experience lived between human beings...a responsible searching, transactional relationships whose meaningfulness demands conceptualization founded on a nurse's existential awareness of self and of the other" (Paterson & Zderad 1976, p. 3). Existential knowing allows us to be concerned with a person's emotional responses to experiences and illness, the understanding of human goals and experiences.

To allow oneself to genuinely or authentically meet "other," to become involved in a "we" relationship, involves persons truly seeking to understand one another. To meet in genuine dialogue or conversation means listening with an "inner ear" or letting the "heart speak." Greene (1984) refers to a "wide-awakeness" or giving full attention to life. The authentic person is able to listen, raise questions, and enter what is said into a sense of newness. An openness with others allows spontaneity and new insights.

In listening to or sharing meaningful experiences, it is the beautiful, the art of nursing that is often heard or told in story form. The meaningful stories are a reminder that the truth does not remain far from us: it can be found in the everyday world of the student and teacher. Together persons experience beautiful moments, and together they ascend the "heights of truth" and are truly authentic. Beautiful moments give meaning to nursing (Paterson & Zderad 1976).

Future Implications for Authentic Living

Beautiful moments or the art in nursing allow persons to see possibilities, to "scale the heights of truth" (Gadamer 1986, p. 15). As

Maxine Greene writes: "It is only when we have in mind a better state of things that we are likely to pay heed to what is lacking in the now and act to surpass it somehow, to get it right" (Greene 1984, p. 13). Individuals may come to recognize what they have potential to be through envisioning possibilities. "I know myself as a being capable of becoming more, capable of actualizing my possibilities. So I am my choices not only in terms of my past but also in regard to my future, my possibilities" (Paterson & Zderad 1976, p. 16).

Nurses who focus solely on accomplishing tasks and performing efficiently, void of an awareness of the humanness of patients and the art in patient-nurse encounters, are, as Gadamer (1986) says: "Souls who...have lost their wings, are weighted down by earthly cares, unable to scale the heights of the truth. There is one experience that causes their wings to grow once again and that allows them to ascend once more. This is the experience of love and the beautiful, the love of the beautiful" (p. 15).

In transcending a view of persons as objects and being more wide-awake, persons may find newness from others' points of view. They come to understand self and others, to "join horizons" or find the "between." The meaning of an other is also "an invitation to new meanings, new ways of Being-in-the-world. The meaning systems of others, their knowledge, is also a source of creativity for us—an invitation to be part of other life forms" (Huebner 1984, p. 122). Encounters of this nature allow for a genuine creation to be made. What happens is not mine or yours but truly ours.

Authenticity thrives in a "we" relationship. As we listen attentively to the other we open the possibility for entering the "play" as described by Gadamer (1976). Gadamer uses the concept of play to provide ontological cues for the way understanding is advanced. He contends that "the basic constitution of the game, to be filled with its spirit—the spirit of buoyancy, freedom and the joy of success" allows the players to enter the dialogue and to be carried by it.

In the following description of a meaningful experience, the student found a reason for Being, the essence of her call into nursing. In the transaction, comfort, joy, and song are the constitution of "play." The patient's strength is shared with the student, providing nourishment to affirm and comfort, to find new understanding in the ability to live and to share joy even during a time of terminal illness and pain.

Going with the visiting nurse to a home visit, this time a convent, and helping with a very long, complicated series of dressing changes was most meaningful. The interaction between the nurse and the patient—so open, so professional, even in the crude environment she worked. I think of this sister quite often—how all her life she gave to others, and now with multiple complications she still finds the strength to joke, sing, converse, and play. She stated to me, "My work is done here on earth. I'm going home 'meaning heaven' for good soon!" It has stayed with me because she had faith still after all this, and I saw the comfort, laughs, and just time this visiting nurse gave. To me this is what nursing should be. (Slunt 1989, p. 136)

The significance of the relationship for both student and patient was the conversation, the sharing that was truly the power behind the meeting. They were united and moved togther, both giving and receiving, creating new meanings. The meaning behind this brief but powerful encounter "stayed with" the student. She received a gift from the patient through humor, song, conversation, and play. In the shared experience, both patient and nurse gave to one another, and the "staying" power remained. The call to authentic compassionate care was fulfilled.

Responsibility in Genuine Encounters

I believe that authenticity means an awareness of care as the foundation of our ethical existence. It calls for a continued struggle to be free. A struggle for freedom means a struggle to be able to reach the patient, to embrace another being with genuine concern. Freedom means reaching beyond the boundaries of the social structure where we often find a resistance to care. It means releasing self from indifference and distancing, a posture often found to exist in an administered bureaucratized society. It means finding real meaning in relationship with another, caring deeply, and affirming caring as a foundation for responsible existence. In the process of caring deeply, persons may be joined together, each caring and being a powerful presence for one another.

We have a responsibility "to help others grow in their own authentic fashions, or to attain a well-being of which they may be deprived" (Greene 1990, p. 30). Pedagogically, this process is more than standing beside students as they discover their dreams, paradoxes, or pain in their calling; it requires risk taking, openness, and trust to be touched by the inner presence of an other.

Being authentic means being open, being willing to engage in self-disclosure. To disclose means to unveil, to make manifest, to show. It means having the courage to Be in the midst of a threat to Being. It means interpreting what is self-disclosed and using that understanding for responsible caregiving. In taking risks, in revealing self, possibilities are openned for more authentic encounters with students and colleagues.

Being authentic as a nurse and educator also creates a tension. There is the dialectic tension of wanting to experience Being but needing to perform doing, or wanting to teach Being but needing to cover content. We have to resist the temptation to build structures, to objectify, if we wish to enter a dialogical, genuine relationship with another. "It is only in changing, uncharted situations that caring acts can be initiated in an authentic sense" (Greene 1990, p. 33).

Since nurses and teachers do not practice in isolation but, rather, are in a profession characterized by interaction and responsibility for others, the definition of authenticity should incorporate the notion of responsibility in the moral-ethical sense. As Levinas (1985) argues, it is the face of the other that compels one to respond, to enter into an ethical, caring relationship. Authenticity in nursing and teaching, then, must take on an ethical, moral, and caring dimension. "Being oneself" is not enough. One may be genuine and sincere but not helpful or therapeutic to a patient or student (Lashley 1990).

Creating a pedagogic presence where conversing, playing, or singing is valued and where authenticity is viewed as the very essence of what it means to care enables students to nurture the authentic voices of persons they are caring for and to more deeply value their own authentic presence with others (Lashley 1990, p. 18). Relating to others in an authentic, yet helpful and therapeutic, manner requires a sensitivity to the places of need within an individual's life. Often caregivers are invited into these places of need. Responding to an invitation to be present to another in a place of need involves receiving the other person, making a commitment to care, and being near at hand to others in distress (Landorf 1984).

An education rooted in authenticity, then, does not simply condone one's right to reveal one's true nature but, rather, engages the student in participating in experiences with others that will shape the authentic persons they are to become. Such an education may also assist students in coming to see themselves as others see them and in developing more sensitivity to the effects of their actions and behaviors on other persons (Lashley 1990, p. 22).

A connection is made with another person in an authentic relationship. Feelings of trust and attachment are fostered. "It is precisely this attachment that forms the basis of a life-giving presence where openness and the transference of positive energy, which affects the other in a profound way, predominates" (Halldorsdottir 1991, p. 44). This mode of "being present" is described as a healing love. The inrush of compassion is like a surge of energy, transformative.

In a professional connection or attachment, there is a space in the between, a space of respect for the other. The nurse cares for the person, but always does this with the intent of letting go, of releasing. Students of nursing may assist patients in shaping the persons they are to become by virtue of an illness experience. Authentic nurses work to make free from dependency those for whom they care. "Nurturing the authenticity of patients is especially important for nurses caring for persons in settings which tend to make patients feel least authentic, such as in highly technological, institutional environments" (Lashley 1990, p. 22). To focus less on skills and more on dialogue is a way to enhance authentic relationships.

With authentic or genuine encounters it is possible to find a balance in relationships, a posture of "being present" or "standing with." Sharing experiences, reflecting upon the uncertainty, anxiety, and hurt associated with being a patient, student, teacher, or nurse helps to illuminate our common bonds, to care responsibly, and to foster authenticity.

References

Benner, P. (1984). *From novice to expert*. Menlo Park, CA: Addison-Wesley.

Caputo, J. D. (1987). *Radical hermeneutics: Repetition, deconstruction, and the hermeneutic project*. Bloomington: Indiana University Press.

Gadamer, H-G. (1986). The relevance of the beautiful. In R. Bernasconi (Ed.), *The relevance of the beautiful and other essays* (N. Walker, Trans.) (pp. 3–53). New York: Cambridge University Press.

Greene, M. (1973). *Teacher as stranger: Educational philosophy for the modern age*. Belmont: Wadsworth.

Greene, M. (1984). Towards wide-awakeness: Humanities in the lives of professionals. In *Literature and medicine: A claim for a discipline*. Proceedings of the Northeastern Ohio Universities College of Medicine's Literature and Medicine Conference.

Greene, M. (1990). The tensions and passions of caring. In M. Leininger & J. Watson (Eds.), *The caring imperative in education* (pp. 29–43). New York: National League for Nursing.

Halldorsdottir, S. (1991). Five basic modes of being with another. In D. Gaut & M. Leininger (Eds.), *Caring: The compassionate healer* (pp. 37–49). New York: National League for Nursing.

Heidegger, M. (1962). *Being and time*. (J. Macquarrie & E. Robinson, Trans.). New York: Harper & Row. (Original work published 1927)

Huebner, D. (1984). The search for religious metaphors in the language of education. *Phenomenology + Pedagogy, 2*(2), 112–23.

Jourard, S. (1971). *The transparent self* (rev. ed.). New York: Van Nostrand Reinhold.

Landorf, J. (1984). *Balcony people*. Waco: Word Books.

Lashley, M. (1989). Being with the elderly in community health nursing: Exploring lived experience through reflective dialogue. (Doctoral dissertation, University of Maryland, College Park). *Dissertation Abstracts International, 51*, 729A.

Lashley, M. (1990, October). *Experiencing the call to care: Creating authentic structures for responsible caregiving*. Paper presented at the Conference on Curriculum Theory and Classroom Practice, Dayton, OH.

Levinas, E. (1985). *Ethics and infinity* (R. A. Cohen, Trans.). Pittsburgh: Duquesne University Press.

Levinas, E. (1987). *Collected philosophical papers* (A. Lingis, Trans.). Boston: Martinus Nijhoff.

Mayeroff, M. (1971). *On caring*. New York: Harper & Row.

Morgan, G. (1983). *Beyond method*. Beverly Hills: Sage Publications.

Neal, M. T. (1989). A room with a view: Uncovering the essence of student experience in a clinical nursing setting. (Doctoral dissertation, University of Maryland, College Park). *Dissertation Abstracts International, 50*, 2847B.

Paterson, J., & Zderad, L. (1976). *Humanistic nursing*. New York: John Wiley & Sons.

Relph, E. (1976). *Place and placelessness*. London: Pion.

Ricoeur, P. (1981). *Hermeneutics and the human sciences*. Cambridge: Cambridge University Press.

Scudder, J. (1990). Dependent and authentic care: Implications of Heidegger for nursing care. In M. Leininger & J. Watson (Eds.), *The caring imperative in education* (pp. 59–66). New York: National League for Nursing.

Slunt, E. T. (1989). Becoming competent: A phenomenological inquiry into its meaning by nursing students. (Doctoral dissertation, University of Maryland, College Park). *Dissertation Abstracts International, 51*, 1196B.

Tillich, P. (1954). *Love, power, and justice.* London: Oxford University Press.

van Manen, M. (1984). Reflections on teacher competence and pedagogic competence. In E. Short (Ed.), *Competence: Inquiries into its meaning and acquisition in educational settings* (pp. 141–58). Lanham, MD: University Press of America.

Watson, J. (1981). The lost art of nursing. *Nursing Forum, 20,* 244–49.

5

Using Lived Experiences to Question Structure and Conformity

Maggie T. Neal

When I encounter the words "structure and conformity as experienced" my neck stiffens. Oddly enough, structure and conformity have always been issues with me... issues that I push against, grapple with, resist, and live within.

Having said that, I must tell you that my life is not chaotic. In fact my life is highly organized and structured in many ways, and in general I conform to the norms of those around me. Why then the bristling at the words? Much of my lived experience as a nurse educator has been within a structure that has not supported my existence as an authentic human being. The experience of living in the communal collective of a technically defined discipline and the grounding of the dominant approach for curriculum planning in the behavioral model do not address the problematic of thinking and acting in situations of difference or uniqueness—situations that are my life existence as a psychiatric nurse and teacher.

I was unable to live authentically within the educational community or the collective world of nursing without feeling that a part of me was dying or that I was becoming homeless. I became marginalized. Only later, and upon reflection, did I begin to question how the prescriptive educational model and the technical reality of the learning environment were contradictory to the caring intention of nursing, the truth-seeking desire of education, and the essential nature of our humanness. This realization caused me to wonder how we could recognize the limits of these theories and practices and move beyond the technical reality they impose on educational practice.

I was led to consider the question, What would an educational community need to be like to initiate, empower, and sustain authentic living in a call to care? Interestingly, that question emerged independently for each of us as we listened to the students' experiences of becoming nurses in the lived curriculum and as we reflected on our own existential situatedness. As we struggled with an expanded view of caring that allows one to be open and aware of possibility and potential, of self-transcendence and a sense of calling, each of us also turned toward ontological issues and the need to extend being into doing and knowing and to extend the ontological into the epistemological. We had to create ways to return to and interpret the more primordial aspects of our calling within the context of being doctoral students pursuing dissertations in clinical settings.

Students Reaction to Structure

In our work with students we have each encountered situations that reflect how current structures negatively affect their ability to care authentically. First, a reflection written by a senior student approaching graduation:

> I track from a distance as my ability to zero specifics is frequently askewed. That is because, from a distance, things don't change very much. While I am acutely sensitive to the aura of my environment, my emotional scope is fairly singular in direction. Thus, I am frequently unable to get a good fix on sources of discomfort.
>
> Recently, however, I was forced to get a little closer to dissect the choices I have made and the reality that shadows them. Nursing school was one choice that brought an upsurge of clipped discomfort in me. I expected humanity to exude from its walls. Instead I encountered highly calculated dehumanization tactics which were under the guise of "behavioral objectives." This strategic staging was perfected to an art form and over the junior year I began to succumb to its force.
>
> Now, as a senior, I have emerged both as a casualty and a survivor. I, too, have become systematic in my approach. I have revamped my expectations and responses to co-exist with the realities of nursing school. Doing so, I have stepped out of the shadows and now feel gusts of warmth. Yet, I wonder what will remain of my original self after I am fully processed through systematic disposal. Perhaps nobody is destined to leave life in his/her original form. Still and all, the process of processing should be approached with caution. What is, in fact, cultivated may (in the end) be self-defeating and pernicious. (Lee 1992)

Perhaps we need to look more critically at the enculturation process that students experience as they enter the world of nursing. "Enculturation" may be defined as appropriating intentional ways of relating to the world (Scudder & Mickunas 1985). It is a process by which one develops structures of meaning for interpreting the world. What historical antecedents and underlying assumptions undergird our educational practices that stress control and conformity, self-estrangement from the professional role to be occupied, and seeing the world through a technical language of behavioral objectives and facts? What compels us to choose a technical way of knowing rather than a knowing grounded in experiences of living? Would it help to enter knowing/learning situations with a shared sense of the moment, inviting students to participate with us in creating an event rather than reducing learning outcomes to behaviors, skills, or facts?

Oliver (1990) makes the distinction between the technical approach to learning, or "knowledge-as-separate object," and the grounded approach to learning, or "knowledge-as-intimate relationship" (p. 67). He argues for "a quality of knowing that is tied, not to an observing mind (somehow located in our heads) and a set of external facts out in the world (as in the old mechanistic Newtonian view), but to the notion of moving both self and becoming-actuality into a common presence, which literally means our sense of feeling before our analytic capacities delineates the object-filled world of preinterpreted things" (p. 68). In this realm of understanding we know and our body understands the significance of the moment prior to our objectifying and interpreting the world—an embodied way of knowing. How do many current curricular structures play a decisive but "voiceless" role in shaping experiences that limit possibilities for knowing/learning?

Through reflection, metaphors written by Mary's students show similar structural concerns that are decisive determinants of students' learning, yet often remain implicit themes in the curriculum horizon:[1]

1. Nursing is like a journey.
   Many choices on the journey have been decided by others.
2. Nursing is like a musical carousel.
   The music is always on a set pace.
   We need to keep a rhythm.
   We find it easy to get caught up in the rhythm.
   Sometimes you are spinning with no beginning or end.
3. Nursing school is like boot camp.
   We lose control of our lives.

4. Nursing school makes us feel like children.
      We are told what to do.
      We aren't given credit for our own thoughts.
      We feel incapable of resuming adult responsibilities.
5. Nursing is like a cult.
      You make us wear these little uniforms.
      We talk the language that you talk.
      We're indoctrinated in the nursing process. (Lashley 1989,
      p. 290)

What happens when the journey of becoming a nurse is highly influenced by others—others who are perceived as having significant control over the students' lives? The students' comments suggest that they are being taught *what* to think and *how* to act rather than *how* to think and *be* in the context of a given moment.

In our work with students we frequently experience a dialectic tension surrounding the need for structure and the resistance to the structure. Because nursing students lack confidence in their ability to "do" nursing, the clinical environment needs structure for them to be somewhat secure, yet it seems to become binding in some way. Emily's students express the vulnerability and tension felt as they encountered the realities of the lived experience of the clinical setting:

- I felt most uneasy about being expected to perform skills on real patients and fear not knowing an answer to a question I'm asked.
- Before you walk into the room to meet your patient you have everything on your mind that you want to do but once you get in there sometimes you get confused.
- Getting used to it: that's a whole new thing, let alone all the complicated procedures. Every day it's just like starting all over again in clinical. (Slunt 1989, p. 2)

How might acknowledging the students' discomfort and the ambiguity of the clinical setting, as well as thinking about meeting each new patient as an "unknown other," help reconceptualize the educational rituals that exist in current curricula? Do we set down too many rules, offer too many guidelines, or make too many assumptions about the absolutes of knowledge and clinical practice? Is that part of what limits one's authentic presence? Given that vulnerability naturally comes with meeting learning challenges, are there better ways to support students throughout their vulnerability? How might we encourage human competence in seeking openness, in risk taking, in asking insightful questions, in meaning making, and in moral and ethical reasoning along with competence in the skills of doing?

The above are but a few examples of the tensions inherent in the way students learn to be nurses. The concerns are repeated often in our work with students throughout the process of becoming nurses. Clearly, it seems that the structural processes of nursing curricula need to be better understood. How might a curricular environment that balances knowing, being, and doing empower students to grapple with issues of structure that estrange them from their primordial call, all within the context of choosing to be with others in situations of illness, caring, and nurturing? What would a curriculum structure look like that encourages vulnerability and allows for greater expression of one's authenticity? How would this change the learning/teaching process?

An Invitation for Transformation

As teachers and researchers, we experience tension between our inherited history of imposing a new curricular structure and the responsibility we feel for inviting students to work collaboratively with us in developing new ways of responding to the call to care through knowing, being, and doing without having a structure externally imposed through our authority. Simply imposing another structure by dogmatic persuasion of the teacher or external control, even when it allows more freedom, only seems to serve a movement causing the pendulum to swing to the other side.

Concern for this notion is heightened by the recent discussion about "curriculum revolution" in nursing (Tanner 1988; Allen 1990; de Tornyay 1990; Moccia 1990; Tanner 1990). Our desire is to move away from the dichotomous thinking that the preexisting structure is inherently "bad" and that any new structure would naturally be better. Rather, we wish to recognize, respect, and critique our historical traditions as we build on them to move our thinking forward and create a transformed future for curriculum theory and nursing practice. Indeed, we believe that it is in the recovering of our past that we may be helped to see beyond present ways of thinking to new possibilities for conceptualizing and structuring nursing and learning experiences that support both vulnerability and authenticity.

In encouraging growth and change, Campbell (1988) suggests that one cannot be creative unless there is willingness to "leave behind the bounded, the fixed, all the rules" (p. 156). That continual leaving, however, is a transformation process, not a revolutionary process. Beittel with Beittel (1991) suggests that "the nature of transformation is radical as opposed to mere change, for in the former something literally becomes something else, a new being grown out of the old" (p. 8). It is not a process that disavows the traditions of the past or rejects its prior experience by going from one kind of half-knowing to another kind of half-knowing. Rather than being a revolution or coup d'état, transformational change proceeds through reflective conversation within a historical context. The focus is not on seeking a new landscape but rather on the experience of having new eyes with which to view or understand better the landscape in which we currently live. The focus is on inner listening to our soul that leads us back to our authentic selfhood and Being-with-others: to our calling. Through the dialectic of sharpening our focus on our inherited landscape and listening to the call from our soul, we can, as Captuo (1986) says, know ourself again. This primordial reacquaintance with our call to care opens possibilities for authentic Being in the presence of others. It potentially leads to taking actions that liberate that which is possible in our situatedness. "Everyone has his specific vocation or mission in life to carry out a concrete assignment which demands fulfillment. Therein he cannot be replaced, nor can his life be repeated" (Frankl 1984, p. 131).

This calling is a challenge for each and every person. Frankl suggests that, rather than questioning the meaning of life, one is questioned by life and must answer to life by being responsible for one's own life. For us then the questions become: In what manner do our own experiences of learning/knowing, structure, vulnerability, and authenticity call us to the caring beings we have always been? How is it we can speak about caring from this place? What allows our speaking from this place to which we have been recalled?

Returning to the Question of Structure

Structure is inherent in any experience, if by structure we mean ways of building, arranging, or fitting together knowledge or experience. Structure, then, seems to imply the ways in which we make meaning of the world around us. Following this line of thinking, Grundy (1987) asserts that curriculum is not an abstract concept. Rather it is a "cultural construction" or a way that one organizes educational practices to show concern for the "experiences people have as a consequence of the existence of the curriculum, rather than with the various aspects which make it up" (p. 6). In other words, one must look with an eye toward the consequences for those involved in the curriculum as lived within a particular communal culture and arising out of a particular historical situatedness.

Using a housing metaphor, Grundy suggests two ways of considering curriculum: conceptual and cultural. In the conceptual approach, one might engage in activities similar to that of a draughtsperson designing a house. One would need to recognize the parameters of basic building design and be responsible for knowing and meeting the minimum requirements of construction for a house as well as the regulations to which such a structure must conform. From there, individual preferences of the client and the client's situation strongly influence the building design. Grundy asserts that the concept of a house and the actions of the house builder are "embedded in the consciousness of the draughtsperson and the expectations of the clients, as well as being embodied in the various regulations to which houses must conform" (p. 5). What are those implicit threads of curriculum drafting to which we need to attend or that we may have forgotten or naively neglected? Would an exploration of curricular rituals allow us to uncover other implicit themes? Where might the notion of calling lead in a curricular sense?

Grundy's cultural view is more concerned with the basic beliefs and values embedded in the way people already live in their place and with the cultural life of the occupant. One would give priority to questions about current practices, preferences, desires, and the social context. Still critical to this view is the need to understand fundamental premises about building design and construction; however, the meaning context has priority. The cultural view, then, points to questions about the ways in which people do and should interact in the world of the lived curriculum. The focus is on relational processes, not structure. How can we understand more directly the beliefs and values critical to being learners, to becoming nurses, to being able to initiate and keep our calling intact in spite of the tendency to forget it because of work structures and distractions of the "everyday"?

In tracing the etymology of the word *structure* one discovers a similar division of the word. Structure may imply a reference to certain features of a building or work, such as those features that are necessary or essential to the building's existence or its basic underlying design, as distinct from those features that complete a work and "bring it into fullness of being" (*Webster's* 1984, p. 787). The underlying structure or supporting framework provides only footings, props, or guides. They are only starting or anchoring points. These specific features, while their presence is clearly acknowledged, are not obviously visible in the completed project.

How might consideration of the underlying structure of experience of the call to care help us more knowingly name what is present in its invisibility? How can we create a supporting ethos of connection, a primary ethic of care/love, and an appreciation for beauty to bound the profession? How could such a structure promote human and technical competence; the vulnerability necessary for openness to life's mysteries, creativity, possibility, and authenticity; and a desire for Being and becoming rather than acceptance of the binding conformity that is so invisibly present? What would happen if these interests were balanced with needed technical interests? How might the structures we create acknowledge our traditions and historical footings as we critically search for innovative ways to transform our practice, whether the practice is education or nursing? What would be required to bring oneself and/or nursing and education into authentic fullness of being? Is there a way to transcend the models of the past without again marginalizing or alienating those who disagree or those who are threatened by change?

Creating a Possible Cultural Horizon for Curriculum

The interpretive framework used in this chapter makes the assumption that understanding the social/cultural world is inherently different from the empirical-analytic approach used to show humans' relation to the natural world. Within such an orientation, the interest is not to discover new universal truths or to propose "grand strategies" that could potentially increase pedagogic certainty and predictability. Rather, the interest here is to give meaning to the encountered pedagogic experiences by uncovering or heightening awareness of the possible meaning structures of lived experiences. The task, however, is not completed by "showing" and "understanding" the subjective dimension of the social/cultural world. The task additionally requires recovering and making explicit the sources of self-knowledge in our biographies and through conversations with others (Darroch & Silvers 1982, p. 17). This is a point to which I will return.

The following Taoist verse invites me to ponder the relevance of curriculum structures by suggesting that it is the connections that we put in place, our understanding of the space we inhabit, and the openings we create for ourselves and others that have fundamental value.

> Thirty spokes share the wheel's hub;
> It is the center hole that makes it useful.
>
> Shape clay into a vessel;
> It is the space within that makes it useful.

Cut doors and windows for a room;
It is the holes which make it useful.

Therefore profit comes from what is there;
Usefulness from what is not there.

(Lao-tzu 1972)

We are reminded to take note that usefulness cannot be thought about in linear terms. Usefulness is like that which calls one to care or calls one into the fullness of Being—to authenticity. Usefulness emerges from the processes of being in relationship with fellow inquirers and patients, from living through experiences of illness and growth, from creating conversational communities, from attending to the primacy of caring in spite of technical and bureaucratic domination, from reflecting and drawing upon self-knowledge, from consciously transforming our understanding of who we are and who we are becoming, and from repeatedly making ourselves vulnerable. And we are asked to remember that usefulness is not in itself enough. We must move beyond usefulness. This is our challenge and our problem to solve.

How then can we appropriate the curriculum—come to grips with the claims of what is explicitly and implicitly there? How can we lay bare the structures of a tradition in such a way that attention is called to our lack of attention to the foundation of the history of our calling? How might our gaze rest on the lived reality in such a way that we can provide adequate phenomenological reconstruction of our situatedness and traditions? Langan (1984) suggests that "appropriation, in the service of authenticity, and authenticity as the quest for the sense of existence, gives phenomenology its direction and meaning and education its mission" (p. 111). This does not take place by happenstance. The stance we take, whether clearly visible, or invisible is still that—a stance.

If the notion of transformation is to be taken seriously, our knowing, while personal, must remain necessarily open in principle and grounded in a contextual public sphere of evolving curricular practices. Understanding that emerges from genuine conversation is not easily compartmentalized. Such knowing moves with one and invites one to advance further. Furthermore, we suggest that our consciousness as curriculum planners needs also to turn to the decisive role that is played by the implicit "horizon" or field surrounding curricula. Given those caveats, we proposed a possible horizon of curricular interests as it emerged from our work with students. It would be a mistake to hold the view that what follows is a grand scheme for

FIGURE 5.1

A Possible Horizon of Curriculum

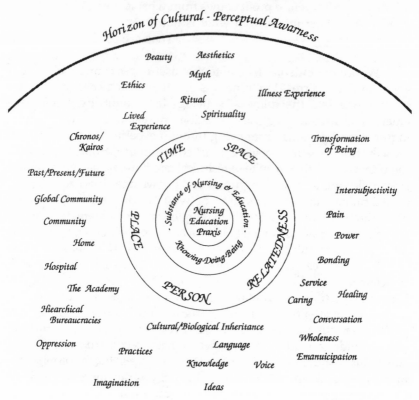

curriculum. The inclusions are momentary assertions representing interests/stances that will no doubt be redefined and changed again as new experiences are encountered (see fig. 5.1).

In thinking about curriculum, we urge that consideration go beyond the tentative model. One might think of the curriculum as a focal model surrounded by a margin or horizon that is a decisive determinate of learning/knowing. The horizon is what makes the unseen factual.

In caregiving professions, we believe that the grounding of a call to Be-in-care is one of the nonfocal aspects surrounding the curricular structure. The notion of curriculum always includes the actual as well as the inactual, the focal and the nonfocal, the thematic and the nonthematic horizon surrounding it. In our inquiry we have shifted our attention from the focal to the nonfocal or perhaps marginal aspect of experiencing the curriculum to make the inactual actual. It is not easy to penetrate the fringe reality of curriculum. Yet, it is only through such scrutiny that lines are found that reach out to the horizon. We have wondered why our abstract conceptions of curriculum have neglected our origins, our beginnings, especially since they are foundational to who we are and the persons we are becoming. Through hermeneutic phenomenology, such a search is possible.

Returning to the Recovery of Self-knowledge

If it is the forgetting of our origins, our beginnings, and the failure of repetition that causes us to not be aware of a sense of calling, then how might such a knowing be sought? Caputo (1986) asserts that we often live our lives "without heeding the transcendental activity that gives shape to our world" (p. 426). He suggests that two tiers of retrieval are always at work and belong together as one goes about the process of repetition. The circle of repetition (the self's recovery of itself) belongs together with the circle of understanding (recovery of the implicit and prethematic). These two circles mirror each other with the ontological (essential) grounding the hermeneutic (methodological). Caputo challenges us to move from our inauthentic fallenness by taking up our authentic potential for Being. He notes that accepting this invitation to take action that liberates the possible requires courage for anxiety and courage for repetition as the self recovers the absence that underlies its presence. Through this process, we recover what we are sent to do and what we are capable of: our forgotten possibility. He points out that "authentically being oneself is the countertendency to inauthentically being like everyone else" (p. 431)—a complaint made by many of our students.

Following a similar line of thought, Beittel with Beittel (1991) suggests that "poetic fragments" and "creative imagination" be used to connect us with the silent mystery of things—"the boundaries of self-other, mind-matter and conscious-unconscious" (p. xv). This work asserts that returning to the "thick of matter" and to the "silent voice of things" for the purpose of renewing consciousness allows "direct contact with the forgotten and disenfranchised things of the world. These things turn out, paradoxically, to be forgotten or undiscovered parts of ourselves and symbols for our unity with the cosmos" (p. xv).

From a structural point of view, how can the curriculum be designed to reveal the process of opening to and/or recapturing a primordial call to Be-in-care? How can this process reveal the hidden as well as the distorted? To what preunderstandings must a student attend in order to recover this understanding? How can one's calling be front and center, be given thematic shape rather than remaining anonymous and prethematic? This naming process, Caputo suggests, is the work of "fetching out" or "laying out" an understanding in which we already stand—a pregiven. It is a knowing that brings us back to what we already know—a knowing again, a renewing of our primordial acquaintance with ourselves. This spiraling process "returns us to ourselves, brings us home. It is appropriation and homecoming: coming into our own again" (1986, p. 434). When successful, this process of self-discovery loosens us from the actual by restoring openness for the mystery of existence as we awaken to our situatedness and penetrate the horizons surrounding us more deeply. It allows us the openness necessary to face the anxiety of realizing our potential for authentic Being (see fig. 5.2).

FIGURE 5.2

Appropriation of Call to Be-in-care

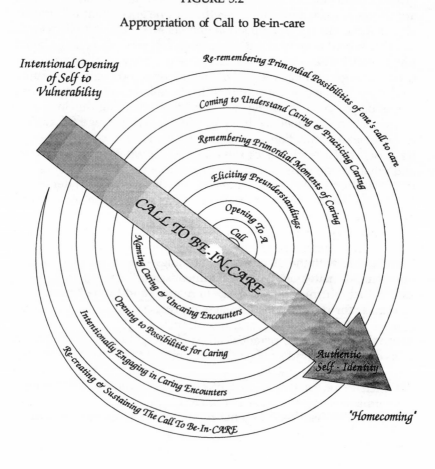

What kinds of curricular processes attend to and support one's intimate remembering and knowing about a call to Be-in-care as one experiences vulnerability in the appropriation of an authentic call? How might reflection become a way of being that promotes the self-distancing necessary to keep open the possibility for authenticity? Given the difficulty in sustaining a call, what might our reflection on our lived experiences of noncaring or irresponsible caring allow us to see? If inauthenticity and rule-bound conformity remain pedagogic and curricular concerns, then would a deconstructive gazing at our caring practices give us the distance and understandings necessary to move beyond the boundaries of caring practices reflected in current curricula?

The Dialectic between Structure and Community

In nursing we have always paid explicit attention to the curriculum that appears on paper and have given less or limited attention to the implicit curricular effects. Traditionally, many of the structural components of the curriculum have been driven by the National League for Nursing guidelines and to a lesser degree by common experiences of the "nursing community." Additionally, the focus on content and technical competence has painfully limited possibilities for knowing/learning and Being. With the recent changes in accrediting practices, perhaps our traditions will become less fossilized and more responsive to the flow and movement of students' learning and the shifting patterns in health care. The questions then become, What does a loss of the former structure allow us to see? What is at stake in a context of more openness? Of more possibility? How might community-building actions support the development of meaningful traditions that reflect our immediate and common experiences? What would happen if we began to imagine ourselves as connected through communities of thought and action instead of being members of educational institutions?

The Context of Current Structure

Through our inquiry we are attempting to understand better the implicit curricular effects as related to issues of vulnerability, authenticity, and structure. To do this we have given attention to the actual lived experiences that structure a student's life and the meaning of those experiences to those living the experiences. We have, through the notion of calling, tried to increase our perceptual awareness of a concern that was previously absent in our consciousness as curriculum planners.

It has been our experience that, as educators, we create structures in nursing to assist students in the process of integrating epistemological knowing. That has been our way of encouraging students to think in logical, rational patterns and to organize vast amounts of nursing knowledge. To that degree our curricula have been successful. However, as we increased the intensity of our gaze on the curriculum, we found ourselves and the students immersed in the language of a technical system that at times results in distancing and alienation of the patient from the nurse. At other times, we found caring constrained by conforming to the systematic, problem-oriented view or the diagnostic view of caregiving. This situation creates a tension between the desire to care for the patient as someone who is unique with dynamic and evolving needs and adhering to predetermined goals and objectives. When nursing is subsumed into the mechanical metaphor of production and efficiency, caregiving takes on a narrow focus; that becomes the focus of student attention as well. Listen again to the voice of a student as she describes her actions: "I went to get my linen before I looked at the patient. Because I want to be organized. And I want her [the teacher] to see that I had set goals and that my AM care is done by nine o'clock. That's how I was thinking. I did not stop to think, 'Maybe the patient needs me to sit and talk to him' " (Lashley 1989, p. 189).

How can we as a nursing community move beyond the unintended rule-bound narratives that have shaped our lives? How might a community need to work through the power structure relations that impact on caring, curriculum, and pedagogy differently from the social structure of a bureaucracy?

Imagining New Contexts for Being

In his work on structure and metastructure, Turner (1969) explores the connections between two models of human interrelatedness. The dialectic between "communitas" (communion of equal individuals) and "social structure" (society as a structured, differentiated, often hierarchical system) is essential for us as individuals and for the societies/institutions in which we live. He notes that in the dialectic "the immediacy of communitas gives way to the mediacy of structure" (p. 129) as one needs to be released from structure to experience communitas and then return to structure revitalized from being in communitas. However, balancing these two experiences is not easy. Because communitas is often rich with pleasurable affects and "life in 'structure' is filled with objective difficulties" (p. 139), the "wisdom is always to find the appropriate relationship between structure and communitas under the *given* circumstances of time and place, to accept each modality when it is paramount without rejecting the other, and not to cling to the one when its present impetuous is spent" (p. 139).

Building on Turner's work, Berman (1988) asserts that social structure implies that persons are seen in terms of positions or through veils such as roles. Social structure keeps an organization going by making laws, institutionalizing language, and stabilizing norms. This analysis seems to describe much of the activity with which nursing has been concerned.

In contrast, communitas is not legislated. "It tends towards spontaneity and wholeness. Social relations are immediate but may not be enduring. Moments are precious and pregnant with possibilities. New forms of communicating and shifting values may be outcomes of communitas. . . In communitas persons probe, see beyond the obvious, and ask increasingly penetrating questions" (p. 302). Communitas has regenerative power that refreshes and is transformative.

Communitas and social structure have differing and discriminating qualities and values (see table 5.1). For example, networks that are loosely connected are quite different from bureaucracies with hierarchial order. Communitas is basically nurturant, emerging from new ideas, new ways of being, genuine mutuality, and power sharing. Structure of social life draws from the riches of power, and persons are often viewed in terms of social, economic, or political positions. Life in structure may be fragmented for the individual, as decisions often are for the good of the organization. Thought and action, which is often concrete, immediate, and ever-changing in communitas, frequently is more abstract and formalized as it becomes institutionalized in the power of social structure. "Social structure provides the language, norms, and glue that sustains society or a group of persons. Communitas is the regenerative power that refreshes a society or group that is the stimulus for change" (Berman 1988, p. 303).

How might we attend to balancing needs for social structure with the experiences of communitas in nursing? How might the development of communitas release persons from their normal settings and thus allow for transformative and creative thinking to reemerge in practice as a result? Turner notes that "structural action swiftly becomes arid and mechanical if those involved in it are not periodically immersed in the regenerative abyss of communitas" (1969, p. 139). What meaning may we take from his injunction?

From a curricular point of view, what is the significance of communitas and social structure? What is the ideal proportion of social structure and communitas? How might notions about communitas help us see different ways of building, arranging, or fitting together

TABLE 5.1

Comparison of Communitas and Social Structure

Characteristic	Communitas	Social Structure
Purpose	Regenerative, speculative, and transformative	Maintenance of order, cohesive, providing "glue"
Values & Norms	Situation specific, relatively rapid rate of change	Concern for universals, slow rate of change
Time Orientation	Of the moment	Rooted in past, extends to the future
Dimensions of Kinship	Matrilineal Bonds "Mother images"	Patrilineal "Father images"
Conception of Person	Wholistic, reflective, caring, mysterious, concern for individual	Role and status oriented, pragmatic, cognitive interest, concern for commonalities
Modes of Thinking	Dialectical, questioning, creative, imagining, personal, immediate	Linear, fragmented, abstract, analytical
Learning/ Knowing	"Sacred" instruction, "spiritual" knowing, ethical knowing	Technical knowledge; legal, political, economic knowledge
Organizational Patterns	Networks, fluid boundaries, equality, person oriented	Bureaucracies, fixed boundaries, hierarchical, task oriented
Decision Making	For good of individual	For good of organization
Level of Affect	Probably high end of continuum	Probably midpoint or below of continuum
Relationship to Pain	Acceptance of pain and suffering	Avoidance of pain and suffering

Adapted from L. M. Berman "Imagining, changing, stabilizing" in T. R. Carson, ed., *Toward a renaissance of humanity: Rethinking and reorienting curriculum and instruction*. (Bloomington: World Council for Curriculum and Instruction, 1988), p. 304.

knowledge, experience, and the meaning making in which we are engaged? Berman (1988) notes that "maintaining communitas involves building and sustaining the inner life through contemplation and imagination. If individuals step back from action to reflection, then creativity can begin to emerge, and persons may have more considered lives to share" (p. 306). Achieving the right balance between structure and communitas would assist us in moving our thinking forward and would encourage the playfulness necessary to connect our ideas with lived reality.

Note

1. The content of the metaphors remains unchanged. Personal pronouns have been made plural and the organization changed for consistency and readability.

References

Allen, D. G. (1990). The curriculum revolution: Radical re-visioning of nursing education. *Journal of Nursing Education, 29*(7), 312–16.

Beittel, K., with Beittel, J. (1991). *A celebration of art and consciousness*. State College, PA: Happy Valley Healing Arts.

Berman, L. M. (1988). Imagining, changing, stabilizing: Maintaining momentum. In T. R. Carson (Ed.), *Toward a renaissance of humanity: Rethinking and reorienting curriculum and instruction.* (pp. 301–12). Bloomington: World Council for Curriculum and Instruction.

Campbell, J. (1988). *The power of myth*. New York: Doubleday.

Caputo, J. D. (1986). Hermeneutics as the recovery of man. In B. R. Wachterhauser (Ed.), *Hermeneutics and modern philosophy* (pp. 416–45). Albany: State University of New York Press.

Darroch, V., & Silvers, R. J. (1982). *Interpretive human studies: An introduction to phenomenological research*. Washington, DC: University Press of America.

de Tornyay, R. (1990). The curriculum revolution. *Journal of Nursing Education, 29*(7), 292–94.

Frankl, V. E. (1984). *Man's search for meaning: An introduction to logotherapy* (rev. ed.) (Ilse Lash, Trans.). New York: Washington Square Press (Original work published 1946).

Grundy, S. (1987). *Curriculum: Product or praxis.* New York: Falmer Press.

Langen, T. (1984). Phenomenology and appropriation. *Phenomenology +
   Pedagogy, 2,* 101–11.

Lao-tzu. (1972). *Tao te ching* (Gia-Fu Feng & Jane English, Trans.). New York:
   Vintage Books.

Lashley, M. E. (1989). Being with the elderly in community health nursing:
   Exploring lived experience through reflective dialogue (Doctoral
   dissertation, University of Maryland, College Park). *Dissertation Abstracts
   International, 51,* 729A.

Lee, S. A. (1992). Class reflections for NURS 418. Undergraduate Program,
   Senior Year. University of Maryland at Baltimore.

Moccia, P. (1990). No sire, its a revolution. *Journal of Nursing Education, 29*(7),
   307–11.

Oliver, D. (1990). Grounded knowing: A postmodern perspective on teaching
   and learning. *Educational Leadership, 19*(6), 64–69.

Scudder, J. R., & Mickunas, A. (1985). *Meaning, dialogue, and enculturation:
   Phenomenological philosophy of education.* Washington, DC: University Press
   of America.

Slunt, E. T. (1989). Becoming competent: A phenomenological inquiry into its
   meaning by nursing students. (Doctoral dissertation, University of
   Maryland, College Park). *Dissertation Abstracts International, 51,* 1196B.

Tanner, C. A. (1988). Curriculum revision: The practice mandate. *Nursing &
   Health Care, 9*(1), 427–30.

Tanner, C. A. (1990). Reflections on the curriculum revolution. *Journal of Nursing
   Education, 29*(7), 295–99.

Turner, V. W. (1969). *The ritual process: Structure and anti-structure.* Chicago:
   Aldine.

Webster's new dictionary of synonyms. (1984) Springfield, MA: Merriam-Webster.

III

Experiencing the Call through Stories in Nursing and Education

What follows are three hermeneutic phenomenological quests. In each, meaning is established through openness to a lived reality that we as nurse educators found ourselves engaged in as we attempted to move beyond the restraints on our way of being with others. Each interpretation reflects how hidden claims made by our technical focus in education and nursing limited our pedagogic practices. Each chapter celebrates the opening of consciousness through the hermeneutic events that claimed our attention. As we entered the world of interpretation, the boundaries of the technical loosened. This opening led to unforseen possibilities, and our interpretation frequently exceeded our conscious intentions.

The inquiry reflects intimate dialogue among students and teachers as partners. From these encounters emerged hidden meanings about a renewed wholeness of being, a new consciousness of caring, and a different perspective of art and beauty. The dialogue brought to the surface new insights about the "in-between" space of what it means to become partners in learning. It became easier to speak of loving students as we opened to the structure of the lived experience—to a call, to care, to Be.

In chapter 6, Mary grapples with questions about being a student of her own practice; particularly, how caregivers are rendered vulnerable and become open to pain as they struggle to find meaning in suffering. Changing her pedagogic approach from learning technical skills and abstract theories to interactive storytelling and reflective dialogue journal writing led to a sense of wonderment and insight about our fundamental relatedness to others. Mary recounts questions that guided her thinking and actions as she restructured learning experiences as students cared for the elderly in their homes.

Concern about the emphasis on a technical definition of competence directs Emily's inquiry in chapter 7 toward a redefinition of caring in the journey toward competence. Turning to inner-world experiences rather than the outer world of observation led her to a deeper understanding of the authentic call to care and the notion of an ever-evolving process of becoming competent. Building on van Manen's notions of pedagogic tact, Emily asks, "How can we make explicit curriculum assumptions as they interface with the personhood of students"?

Drawing on Gadamer's inquiry of art and aesthetic consciousness, Maggie wonders what it would be like to consider a student as a work of art in creation as she askes, What does it mean to undergo an experience with a group of students? How are experiences of "the beautiful" and caring similarly grounded? In chapter 8 she describes how reflective writing and reciprocal conversation illuminate the experience of learning to give nursing care and how a call to nursing comes into being.

6

Being with the Elderly:
A Unique Call to Care

Mary Ellen Lashley

The experiences I have had teaching nursing students have led me to raise questions about my own practice. I have wondered how I could inspire students to reach beyond the limitations of their present perspectives without negating or ignoring the inherent worth and dignity of their personal histories. In what ways did the structure of a formal undergraduate nursing curriculum promote freedom of inquiry and exploration? Were there ways in which it snared persons, leaving some too tightly grasped and others crushed and broken? Questions such as these led me to pursue my doctoral dissertation research within the context of my own teaching practice.[1] In this chapter, I discuss the process I went through in my research as I explored the questions that emerged for me in my own inquiry and the context in which my research unfolded. The chapter also highlights the approach I took in response to these questions and the insights I derived from questioning and reflecting on a shared learning experience with my students.

How I Came to the Question

As a nurse educator, I find that my students seem to struggle to find meaning in the midst of human suffering. I have wondered how I could provide opportunities for students to seek personal relevance and to create meaning as they uncover a deeper understanding within their nursing experiences. Would it be possible for students to come to view my authority in a different manner? Could students come to recognize their responsibility in contributing to their learning experience? Could we establish a sense of community that is based upon intrinsic felt commitments toward others rather than on a sense of domination or external control?

As I pondered these questions, I also wondered whether I would find comfort in valuing the experiences of others and in letting go of some of the control I exercised in structuring the learning experience. What would it be like to be confronted with the very real gaps in my own understanding by participating in a shared learning experience with my students? What structures would permit authentic self-disclosure in a manner educationally meaningful to all participants? What would be the implications of disclosing and making manifest the origins of our own personal calls to care?

Questions such as these made me acutely aware of my own vulnerability and yet filled me with a sense of wonderment as I saw myself evolving as a person through this process of reflection and inquiry. It was questions such as these that prodded me to move forward in my thinking and inquiring about what it meant to be "called to care."

As I contemplated how to assist students to find meaning in suffering, I was attracted to an unusual distinction between the meaning of problems and questions. For example, Burch (1986) delineates a difference between stating a problem and raising a question. Burch's writing, I believe, may be helpful to those who find themselves asking the kinds of questions that I struggled with. Burch notes that problems concern objects or things which are set off from oneself. Questions, on the other hand, pertain to one's very Being. They are subjective, indeterminate, and elude certainty. One does not so much posit a question as one is encompassed by it. Finally, problems are attacked using predetermined methods with the goal of seeking resolution and finding closure. Questions, on the other hand, do not seek a definitive answer but, rather, seek to understand more fully the context in which the question arises (Burch 1986).

In my inquiry, I found that I could state a discrete problem and follow it through with a technical approach, but this research approach did not seem to adequately capture what I was wondering about. Questions, however, seemed to emerge naturally from reflection on my experiences as they were lived. While these questions captured more accurately my wonderings, they eluded my attempts to find definitive answers. At the same time, however, they brought clarity to the broader context in which my questions arose.

Looking at the notion of questions and problems from a more philosophical, phenomenological perspective meant a departure from the psychological lens I had used to define problems. A psychological orientation to problems presupposes an ultimate goal of finding answers and, in so doing, may mask the deeper philosophical meanings inherent in the questions themselves.

The broader notion of questioning is in keeping with the work of van Manen (1991), who views problems encountered in teaching as situations, predicaments, or possibilities: "Ultimately predicaments and difficulties constitute 'problems of meaning,' or rather questions of meaning...Meaning questions cannot be 'solved' and done away with once and for all...difficulty is something we have to interpret, work at, and remain attentive to" (p. 107–8).

Lee (1989) also speaks to this notion when she differentiates between well-structured problems, which are linear and sequential and lend themselves more readily to analytic rules for arriving at a single correct solution, and life's more "wicked" problems, which are ill structured and context dependent and are dealt with through multiple lenses and approaches. In nursing, it is these wicked problems that tend to confront one's practice on a daily basis.

The Context in Which Questions Emerged

My research unfolded in the context of a community health clinical nursing experience in which students visited and cared for elderly persons in their homes. By sharing personal life stories and reflecting on significant nursing experiences, the students and I disclosed the meaning of this particular clinical experience.

As we cared for elderly persons in their homes and communities, we were committing to a relationship that rendered us vulnerable and open to experiencing pain. In addition, by becoming an inquirer into my own presence in teaching, I became in essence a student, studying and learning about my practice. Changing the structure of the curriculum experience in this way was unsettling for both me and the students. I was rendered vulnerable as I became more consciously aware of the meaning of our experience and of the stories that we were telling to one another and living out together.

Changing the way we structured our experience also required that I look at my practice in a different light. If personal voice and experience become a point of departure for learning about a clinical experience, what would happen to the content I felt so necessary to cover in this course? On the other hand, when "content" is devoid of "context," what relevance does it have? How could I maintain a therapeutic presence with students without moving into the realm of therapy, which lies beyond my pedagogic commitment? In my doctoral dissertation I reflected on this painful struggle:

> I knew that this curriculum experience would demand honesty toward my students. I was not sure I was prepared to deal

with the depth of honesty required of me...Throughout my journey, I experienced both existential and psychological anguish. The psychological anguish emerged as I came to know students as persons and began to experience the grief, loneliness, and loss they had faced in the existential moments of their lives...The existential anguish I experienced in this study was manifested in the struggle I felt between my intense desire for completion and the uncertainty I felt knowing that there was no guarantee that the completion I sought would be valuable once it was achieved. (Lashley 1989, pp. 260–62)

Was it possible for me to share in and yet stand apart from another's pain? How could being moved by another's distress promote an involvement that relieved the person in need from the burden of carrying a distress alone but did not incapacitate me in the process? Could I experience closeness with my students without being submerged by this involvement?

Gadamer (1975) contends that questions of meaning often arise in the midst of negative or painful life experiences. Greene (1973) refers to these experiences as encounters with absurdity. These are experiences from which arise questions that have no answers. In nursing, we are constantly confronted with these kinds of experiences. Therefore, I found myself asking, How can students come to find meaning in these experiences? It became clearer that the kinds of questions that I was surfacing about my practice would require that I talk about nursing in a different way.

As I continued on this journey to understand more fully the meanings of student experiences, I chose hermeneutic phenomenology as a point of departure. I found this perspective helped foster an alternative paradigm for my inquiry. Experiencing a clinical setting phenomenologically necessitated that the students and I examine the personal meaning that these experiences held for us and for others entrusted to our care. By valuing their own authentic persons, the students were able to speak freely from their own experiences and came to value their unique contribution in authoring the clinical experience. In essence, they experienced the call to care through the extension of their most authentic selves.

Nursing as an Extension of Being

In this clinical experience, the students and I attempted to view the cognitive and psychomotor dimensions of nursing as an extension of our Being. Rather than separating our facts and skills from who we were as persons, we started by developing our voices and by speaking through personal experience. Broader, more abstract, theoretical notions, however, arose out of reflection on concrete experience.

This approach to practice required that we talk about nursing differently; that is, by using personal autobiographies and stories as a point of departure for theorizing about and practicing nursing. Since necessary facts and skills relevant to our practice were viewed as extensions of our being, the focus changed from technical skills and abstract theoretical notions to autobiography, storytelling, and reflective dialogue. These stories provided a context to discuss meaningfully content related to aging and skills necessary to minister to the needs of older persons. Essentially, the students and I dialogued about significant past and present life experiences that shaped our perception of and response to the clinical experience.

Creating Meaning through Narrative

As we engaged in a home-visiting experience with the elderly, we reflected on the meanings of our experiences through oral and written conversation. Written conversation took the form of dialogue journal writing. Dialogue journals are an interactive and responsive form of communication in which students and teacher carry on an ongoing conversation as they share their feelings and experiences in writing (Staton 1987). In the dialogue journal, the teacher has an opportunity to respond to students' individual needs, provide reassurance and support, and challenge them to move beyond their present level of understanding by presenting new ideas and by questioning existing preconceptions (Staton 1987).

The interactive nature of both oral and written reflective dialogue enabled us to integrate domains of personal experience and consequently realize new meanings and insights that transcended individual understanding. The dialogue also nurtured a sense of community between persons by providing the opportunity for my students and me to participate in dialogue, as, together, we authored the experience and brought meaning to it.

I created my text for analysis by recording and transcribing our oral and written conversations. My reflections on the major themes emerging from the texts produced by this interactive discourse were brought back to the students for continued dialogue and reflection. This process of reflection involved sharing our experiences, analyzing the assumptions and prior understandings on which our perceptions of our experiences rested, examining the sociohistorical context in which experiences unfolded and finding coherence, integrity, pattern, and form among the great diversity represented by our experiences (Vandenborn 1982).

Emerging Themes

The major themes of place, presence, and authenticity were disclosed as a common ground of the experience of caring for the elderly. (Examples of how these themes emerged in the students' written descriptions are illustrated in table 6.1. Key words or phrases which point to these central themes are underlined.)

TABLE 6.1

Excerpts from Written Descriptions

Place
1. Entering strange *homes* in unfamiliar *settings* is frightening.
2. I'm terrified of the *city*.
3. I need to feel secure in my *surroundings*.
4. Entering the *home* made me sick to my stomach.
5. The client was in a *dark room* which was frightening.
6. I'm terrified of what is behind the *door*.

Presence
1. *Being present* may be the greatest strength I bring to nursing.
2. I felt *present* with a patient who had suffered a stroke and could not speak. I *stayed with* the patient, held her hand, and explained what was happening.

Authenticity
1. Old age is like an old safe.
   What is *inside* is always a mystery.
   The *contents* are precious.
   The elderly have value in their *experience* which is waiting to be found.
2. Old age is like winter.
   People stay *inside* where it's warm. When *outside*, you may never know someone's home.
   Like an old person's appearance and their *actual self*—How they are *inside*.
3. Old age is like an old book.
   A book's value is *individual*.
   A book represents *different experiences and life stories*.

Place

Maintaining self-esteem and integrity while being with patients on their own "turf" created many challenges for my students. Threats to physical and emotional well-being were unmasked in students' expressions of concern for their physical safety, statements of tension in being on "someone else's turf," and the desire to return to their familiar home ground of the hospital institution. Students expressed feelings of vulnerability in losing control of the physical places they shared with their patients.

However, the vulnerability that students experienced in the home created a tension that prodded them to venture forward and come to know the significance of these places in the lives of their older patients, to know the symbols in homes that were powerful in revealing important aspects of the patient's life story, and to recognize that meanings stem not only from places but also from one's own experiences and interpretations (Relph 1976).

While students perceived the hospital setting as a place where their presence was accepted, they seemed to perceive the home as a place where their presence was viewed as intrusive. In the following excerpt, we reflect on the differences experienced when being with persons in these two unique places where nursing care is given.

Tracy: I think, in the hospital, you're expected to be there as a nurse...That's a common role. But the home, you're not...

Mary: How does the home space differ from other spaces that we occupy in life?

Natalie: You let down your barriers...

Rachael: It's your personal place. Where nobody else really has a right to come in and look into your drawers and go in your closets...

Mary: As nurses, how can we reverence another person's space? Do you think that it requires a greater sensitivity when you're in the home?

Jean: You have to feel comfortable and they have to feel comfortable in your home. I think once you do feel comfortable in their home, you can do a lot more. But if you feel you're always an outsider,...you can always try and try and it's just difficult. (Lashley 1989, p. 137)

Jean's statement of feeling as though she were an outsider reveals a dimension of Being in which one stands outside or inside the experience of place. Relph (1976) identifies an "insider" as a person who normally lives within the place or environment being studied. "The insider's world is grounded in the everyday experience of living in a particular environment; it involves processes and events normally unnoticed and unquestioned" (Seamon 1984, 130–31). Places may have meaning to the degree one falls inside that place (Relph 1976). Being "inside" a place involves a feeling of enclosure and security rather than a feeling of being threatened or exposed (Relph 1976).

The deepest experience of place is felt when one is "existentially inside" an experience. Existential insideness involves a sense of belonging, of identity, and of commitment to the place being occupied. The place is felt as part of oneself (Relph 1976).

The home place is a profound center of human existence where persons may dwell as existential insiders. The home place is foundational to one's identity as an individual and as a member of a larger community. The home is an irreplaceable center of significance in one's life and a point of departure from which one derives one's orientation and position in the world (Relph 1976). In this study, the elderly persons cared for were the existential insiders to the home ground where care was given.

Persons may also dwell "empathetically inside" an experience. Empathetic insideness is a "situation where a person who is an outsider in terms of place works through concern, interest, and empathy to understand that place and come to know its essential meaning and structure" (Seamon 1984, p. 132). Empathetic insideness requires a willingness to be open to the significance of a place in the life of another, to know and respect the symbols within places, to understand that a place is rich in meaning, and to recognize that meanings stem not only from places but also from one's own experiences (Relph 1976). In this study, students experienced the call to be empathetic insiders.

Facilitating an aging person's sense of place required an environment where persons had choices over their lives and could be surrounded by those things that were personally meaningful to them. Elderly persons, rendered vulnerable by illness or injury, are often comforted by surroundings that foster continuity and preserve a coherent sense of self-identity. Entering the home and sharing family stories, pictures, and memorabilia enabled the student to experience the patient's world, to go beyond superficialities, and to become involved with the person on a deeper level. Older persons were encouraged to find meaning in their lives through reflection on past life experiences. This type of therapeutic reminiscence was nurtured in the context of the patient's home, where persons were surrounded by those things that held greatest meaning for them. As such, the home provided a supportive environment where students learned the significance of the places they shared with persons they cared for and where they could value their presence by "Being with" those entrusted to their care.

Presence

Embodied in the notion of presence is the idea of being in sight or near at hand (Skeat 1882). Students seemed to struggle with their patients' desires to have them care for them by simply "Being present." While they experienced the tension between "Being with" and "doing for" the patient, the elderly patient communicated the value of Being present by requesting their continued presence in the home and by valuing their presence despite limited hands on physical care. Monica disclosed this dilemma in the following journal entry:

> I have mixed feelings about working with this client. Some days I feel very frustrated and question whether I am truly able to help her. I feel as if she is not listening to anything I say. I often wonder where her mind is when I'm *talking to* her. At other times, I feel as if maybe just *being there* for a visit and *being a good listener* is what she needs the most. She seems to need someone to *talk with* her so she doesn't feel so alone and isolated. Sometimes, she repeats something I said the week before and this makes me realize that she must hear some of what I say. (Lashley 1989, p. 144)

The concern that "I am not learning or *doing* anything" reflected the struggle students face in laying aside their technical skills and information giving roles and valuing their physical and emotional presence with others. Natalie wrote:

> While preparing to write in my journal, I began to think about the word caring and how sometimes it seems that when people talk about "nursing care of patients" or "caring for patients"—they mean the physical aspects of *taking care of* someone, rather than the emotional *"caring for"* someone. (Lashley 1989, p. 144)

My students found that to be present with the patient required great personal sacrifice in order to overcome the time limitations imposed by the organization. Great value was placed on the ability of systems to run efficiently. The place of caregiving assumed a narrow focus when viewed from this type of mechanical metaphor.

At times, caring was constrained by conforming to a systematic, problem-oriented view of caregiving. This condition created a struggle between the desire to be present to others and the pressure of adhering to static, prearranged goals and objectives. Rachael sensed this tension as she attempted to set goals for planning care on a medical unit:

> I went to get my linen before I looked at the patient. Because I want to be organized. And I want her [the teacher] to see that I had set goals and that my AM care is done by nine o'clock. That's how I was thinking. I did not stop to think "Maybe the patient needs me to sit and talk to him." (Lashley 1989, p. 189)

Kate recounted a similar story as she experienced the tension of putting the need to be present with her patient and family ahead of conforming to daily, preset objectives:

> I had spent some time maybe half an hour, talking to the mother. Which I felt was really necessary. But in the end it ended up putting me a bit behind...And in the back of my mind this little voice is saying..."You shouldn't have spent time with that mother. You should have stuck to your goals and objectives for the day. You should have finished your work." (Lashley 1989, pp. 189–90)

Authenticity

Nurturing authenticity was a vital thread in my students' ideal of what it meant to be present with their elderly patients in the home. The term *authenticity*, encompasses the notion of being real or genuine. The theme of authenticity was particularly evident in the metaphors students created to depict their perceptions of the experience of old age (see table 6.1).

In addition, my students often expressed concern over the loss of their own sense of self that was felt by being consumed in the nursing role. Their conversation echoed a feeling of powerlessness and vulnerability and a loss of a sense of self-identity. The metaphor of nursing as a cult poignantly illustrated their feelings of loss of self-identity. As Kate noted:

> You know what I really think...I think nursing is a cult...Because you get us in here and you indoctrinate us with all this nursing process. And you make us wear these little

uniforms...And talk this language that you talk. And then you
send us out...to get more people in. (Lashley 1989, p. 191)

Tracy expressed concern over her teacher's admonition that "You
will be conformed to our framework...of this institution of nursing"
(Lashley 1989, p. 192).

I knew...that means that...what they are going to be
teaching me is the way that I'm going to be changing...If I want
to go through this curriculum, I need to accept that...Because
if I don't conform to it, I'll be out. And you can't...go through
this curriculum without conforming an awful lot. (Lashley 1989,
p. 192)

These comments are in keeping with the contention that we
cannot become transparent in our language, because our cultural
traditions and networks of causal relations influence our ability to
exercise individual choice (Street 1992). I wondered, then, how I,
together with my students, could work out a structure that fostered a
greater sense of relatedness and authenticity rather than impose a
preexisting structure that contributed to a sense of alienation. How
could persons come to an understanding of the knowledge, skills, and
abilities necessary to practice professional nursing without losing a
sense of themselves as unique persons in the process? What could be
done to bring us back in touch with our original call to care, that which
compelled us to enter into a profession of responsible caregiving? How
could students come to value the contributions they each brought to
the profession because of their unique life stories? And finally, what
was the impact of my pedagogic presence in creating supportive
environments that nurtured the dialogue that allowed these types of
questions to be brought to disclosure?

It seemed as though a new structure needed to be created to allow
greater expression of the authentic person. Still, as teacher and
researcher, I was torn between my own interest in imposing a new
structure and the responsibility I felt to encourage my students to
collaboratively develop a new way of fitting together ways of knowing,
being, and doing in nursing without having a structure externally
imposed by my authority. I did not wish to simply impose another
structure by dogmatic persuasion or external control. I also wished to
move away from the dichotomous thinking that the preexisting structure
was inherently "bad" and that any new structure would naturally be
better. Rather, I desired to recognize and respect our historical traditions,

building on them to move forward in our thinking about nursing theory and practice. I felt that it was in the recovering of our past that we might be helped to see beyond present ways of thinking to new possibilities for conceptualizing nursing.

Since nurses practice not in isolation but, rather, in a profession characterized by interaction and responsibility for others, it seemed to me that, in nurturing an authentic presence with students, I could not overlook the aspect of authenticity that incorporated the notion of responsibility or the moral-ethical sense embodied in Greene's (1973) definition of authenticity as the sense of the person one *ought* to be. As Levinas (1985) argues, it is the face of the other that compels one to respond and to enter into an ethical relationship. Authenticity in nursing, then, must take on an ethical or moral dimension. To be human is to be conscious and to be responsible. Since every moment holds with it numerous possibilities, when one chooses one course of action, the other possibilities are condemned to nonbeing. Still, what is chosen is born into the world because of one's decision and is forever preserved from nonbeing. Despite restrictions in one's environment, persons retain this freedom to give some shape to their existence and their destiny (Frankl 1963). Responsible caring, then, seems to involve the caregiver in assisting persons to become responsible for their own lives, choices, and decisions (Mayeroff 1971). Caregivers, whether teachers, nurses, or students, may assist those cared for to find meaning in their experiences by helping them to see their responsibility for realizing the many possibilities inherent within their existence (Frankl 1963).

To grow as a person is to transform choices into commitments and to become responsible for one's choices (van Manen 1991). To nurture self-responsible maturity, one must develop a tactful way of Being (van Manen 1991). Tactful action is oriented to the good of the other and seeks to protect what is vulnerable. Tactful actions seek to prevent hurt, heal what is broken, strengthen what is good, enhance what is unique, and sponsor personal growth. To accomplish these goals, a "speech climate" must be created that is personal, relational, and situation specific, one that does not conform to rigid, set rules for dialogue. This speech climate must also be moderated by silence and supportive nonverbal communication and be lived out through example (van Manen 1991).

It seems as though much of the language currently in use to express the technical, interpretive, or critical orientation to a dialogue on caring is alienating. The language of technique has been criticized for being too objective and devoid of a personal voice. The language of critical inquiry presupposes a hermeneutics of suspicion and tends to place social problems in the context of power relations. The language of interpretive inquiry has been criticized for a lack of attention to oppressive forces that shape the context in which questions for inquiry emerge. Is it possible to communicate through a language that clearly and sensitively reflects the conflicts and tensions inherent in the world of nursing? If so, it would seem that this language would need to allow for the expression of ideas related to ethics, community, and responsibility and would emerge from the real life experiences of persons as they engage in reflection on practice.

Implications for Being Called to Care

As a nurse educator and a researcher into my own practice, I came to discover that the insights and experiences shared with my students were enhanced by allowing our questions to move us in new directions for making meaning of our experiences. Initially, it was our own personal life stories that enabled us to recognize our fundamental relatedness to others. Creating a pedagogic presence where the sharing of personal life stories were valued and where authenticity was viewed as the very essence of what it meant to care enabled the students to nurture the authentic voices of persons they were caring for and to more deeply value their own authentic presence with others. It was equally important, though, to interpret what was self-disclosed and to use the information for responsible caregiving and professional action (Jourard 1964).

Even, at times, when students' authentic presence could be viewed as unprofessional or inappropriate, these behaviors were examined from a perspective rooted in relatedness and authenticity. By standing side by side (Scudder & Mickunas 1985), we could examine the incident together, taking into consideration what it might be like to experience the patient's world. For example, older persons may struggle with feelings of dependency. By reflecting with students on their own personal experiences with dependency, helpful ways of being with others experiencing these feelings could be illuminated. Students would then validate responsible actions for caregiving by opening up dialogue with patients on the meaning of these experiences and the perceived helpfulness of nursing responses. Such a response to caregiving served to extend the students' empathic boundaries (Travelbee 1966). Students were also assisted in examining the sociohistorical contexts in which these experiences were interpreted. In this way, my students were encouraged to take an active role in structuring the experience. Ultimately, they came to sense their responsibility to create a therapeutic presence with patients and a meaningful, personally relevant, and collaborative pedagogical experience with others. Since this experience, I have wondered whether to begin the next clinical experience with the profound quote by Buber: "There is no responsibility unless there is one to whom one is responsible" (Glatzer 1966, p. 21). Together, we could explore what it means to be responsible in nursing and to whom we are responsible.

Travelbee (1966) asserts that to use oneself therapeutically requires a commitment to the other and an affirmation of the other as a unique and irreplaceable individual who is unlike any other person. When one experiences the privilege of encountering another human being, one may appreciate the miracle of having another person "near at hand."

The findings of my study seem to point to the importance of creating an environment that nurtures authenticity. For elderly patients, reminiscing on past events may enable them to transcend the immediate location and to participate in past experiences. The elderly person, then, is freed to dwell in places evoked through reminiscence. Since, with aging, persons may experience progressive limitation of activity, this manner of participating in past places and events may assist persons to express themselves as unique individuals, to find meaning in their experiences, to transcend immediate limitations and restrictions, and to rediscover a forgotten sense of coherence in personal identity (Godkin 1980).

The students' abilities to surrender control of the environment and to enter into the home of the elderly also allowed them to view the aging individual as a unique person living in a distinct social and cultural context. Providing opportunities where persons could voice what was personally meaningful to them in the context of their own worldviews facilitated authenticity for both students and patients. Institutional and time constraints that impede the nurse's ability to nurture the voice of the patient as a unique person need to be explored and acted upon. Nurses need to create conditions and places in which it is possible to value authenticity in both themselves and others.

In the context of nursing education, more emphasis may need to be placed on creating a context to prepare nurses to care by providing opportunities for students to seek personal relevance, create meaning, and understand dimensions of human experience through shared experiences and relationships (Roderick 1988). Engaging in reflective dialogue may enhance participants' self-awareness and understanding and may enable participants to envision new possibilities for caring for the elderly. Reflective dialogue may also provide integration of the student's and teacher's personal experience, resulting in the realization of new meanings and insights transcending individual understanding. The dialogue may also nurture a sense of community between persons by providing the opportunity for students and teacher to become participants in dialogue, as they author the experience and bring meaning to it.

In this study, meaning was facilitated by grounding students' experiences with the families under their care in their own personal life stories and events. Reflection on the problems and needs facing students' own families of origin served as a point of departure in helping them to surface ethical dilemmas in the families under their care and broadened their vision of the complex, multidimensional issues facing the aging population. In this way, the clinical experience was transformed into a personally relevant and collaborative pedagogical experience. In addition, by supporting their elderly patients' attempts to share their family stories, students were better able to see each patient as a human being in meaningful relationships with others and within the context of a larger society.

Transforming Curriculum through Dialogue

Through extensive writing and discussion, the lives and stories of teachers and students may be brought to disclosure. These stories, discussions, and personal biographies serve to inform and reform educational practices. Both teacher and student take a dynamic and collaborative stand in continually recreating the curriculum (Meath-Lang 1989).

The themes emerging from the stories and discussions in this study seemed to possess a transformative dimension as the students and I began to explore, in addition to the traditional curriculum threads, the experience from curriculum themes grounded in lived experience. In a sense, we became cocreators in developing our own conceptual lens for making meaning of the world around us. The students, then, not only were involved in application of a conceptual model but actually contributed to the creation of an alternative philosophical perspective. The aim of this endeavor, however, was not to generalize my findings by suggesting the adoption of themes revealed in this study into a structured curriculum for nursing but to appropriate the meanings of the experience into individual lives and to expand the vision of what it meant to be with and care for the elderly.

In addition to the changes in thought produced by this discourse, changes in actions toward others were also evidenced. Gradually, the students moved toward developing a "community of otherness" (Arnett

1986). This community of otherness was characterized by recognition that we all shared a common concern and a common situation but approached the situation differently, depending upon our unique experiences and traditions. While we attempted to move toward equalization of power relationships and affirmation of persons apart from roles, we came to recognize that this movement did not, in itself, guarantee community. To work out problems in relationships required a shift from control to dialogue, from image to authenticity, from independence to interdependence, and from prescription to collaboration (Arnett 1986).

Buber notes that to be an "ethical community" requires being willing to label the shortcomings in a community. Since no community is ideal, persons strive for freedom to engage in critical scrutiny, promotion of egalitarian ideals, and movements between different communities to maintain openness. Freedom involves a tension between critiquing and preserving the structure of a community (Arnett 1986).

In this experience, freedom was restrained to a degree to avoid anarchy. However, rather than prescribing a specified framework for the call to care, students were pointed in a direction of responsible caring through storytelling and narrative. These narratives were then offered for review and critique. As Buber notes, narrative permits an encounter with freedom through recognition of one's own uniqueness (Arnett 1986).

This patterning of freedom through community was also reflected in students' interactions with those entrusted to their care. Students allowed more time for patients to share their own stories and to explore with them patterns of meaning within their human experiences. Sensitivity was demonstrated in nonverbal communication by the use of silence, attentive posturing, and attending to the "face of the other." Persons moved toward the ideal of "tactful action" (van Manen 1991) by attempting to relate from the patient's point of view, and by not imposing their own sense of understanding onto the patient. A greater focus was placed on creating a place in the home to nurture the patient's life story to disclosure.

The experience also enabled participants to see both the similarities and the disparities between the traditional conceptual model governing the curriculum and the views borne out of lived experience. In addition, by creating an environment where students could search together for meaning in their experiences, a heightened sense of community and responsibility for others were nurtured. Students came to see their responsibility and their value to the group in bringing meaning to the experience by sharing their unique perspectives and by questioning and reflecting upon their own traditions.

When one reasons through dialogue, new patterns of knowing are discovered that assist in the creation of a new understanding. It is through this creative endeavor that the art of nursing is expressed. "Art joins dissimilar experiences by finding the image that unites them at some deeper emotional level of meaning" (Younger 1990, p. 41). This recognition of pattern, form, or fit fills gaps in one's experience.

Through my research, themes of place, presence, and authenticity were disclosed as a common ground of the lived experience of nursing students who were caring for older persons in their homes. Each theme was examined for its potential in generating new possibilities for nursing practice and education and for raising new questions for continued dialogue and reflection. The insights derived through reflective dialogue and conversation created a structure for making meaning of the experience which was rooted in collaboration and personal relevance and which nurtured a sense of responsibility for the growth and development of self and others.

Note

1. This work is based on: Lashley, 1989. Research for this project was made possible in part by a grant from the Faculty Research Committee at Towson State University.

References

Arnett, R. (1986). *Communication and community: Implications of Martin Buber's dialogue.* Carbondale: Southern Illinois University Press.

Burch, R. (1986). Confronting technophobia: A topology. *Phenomenology and Pedagogy, 4,* 3–19.

Buttimer, A., & Seamon, D. (Eds.). (1980). *The human experience of space and place.* London: Croom Helm.

Darroch, V., & Silvers, R. J. (Eds.). (1982). *Interpretive human studies: An introduction to phenomenological research.* Lanham: University Press of America.

Frankl, V. E. (1963). *Man's search for meaning: An introduction to logotherapy* (rev. ed.) (Else Lasch, Trans.). New York: Washington Square Press. (original published 1946).

Fulwiler, T. (Ed.). *The journal book.* Portsmouth: Boynton/Cook.

Gadamer, H-G. (1975). *Truth and method.* New York: Crossroad.

Glatzer, N. (Ed.). (1966). *The way of response: Martin Buber.* New York: Schocken Books.

Godkin, M. (1980). Identity and place: Clinical applications based on notions of rootedness and uprootedness. In A. Buttimer & D. Seamon (Eds.), *The human experience of space and place* (pp. 73–85). New York: St. Martins Press.

Greene, M. (1973). *Teacher as stranger: Educational philosophy for the modern age.* Belmont: Wadsworth.

Jourard, S. (1964). *The transparent self.* Princeton: D. Van Nostrand.

Lashley, M. E. (1989). Being with the elderly in Community Health Nursing: Exploring lived experience through reflective dialogue (Doctoral dissertation, University of Maryland, College Park). *Dissertation Abstracts International, 51,* 729A.

Lee, D. (1989). Everyday problem solving: Implications for education. In J. Sinnott (Ed.), *Everyday problem solving: Theory and application* (pp. 251–65). New York: Praeger.

Levinas, E. (1985). *Ethics and infinity: Conversations with P. Neno* (R. A. Cohen, Trans.). Pittsburgh: Duquesne University Press.

Mayeroff, M. (1971). *On caring.* New York: Harper & Row.

Meath-Lang, B. (1989). The dialogue journal: Reconceiving curriculum and teaching. In J. Peyton & D. Jurich (Eds.), *Perspectives on journal writing: Students and teachers write together* (pp. 3–17). Washington, DC: TESOL

Peyton, J. & Jurich, D. (Eds.). *Perspectives on journal writing: Students and teachers write together,* Washington DC: TESOL.

Relph, E. (1976). *Place and placelessness.* London: Pion.

Roderick, J. (1988). Peer dialogue communities: Recreating the curriculum. *Dialogue, 5*(2), 15–16.

Scudder, J. R., & Mickunas, A. (1985). *Meaning, dialogue, and enculturation: Phenomenological philosophy of education.* Washington, DC: Center for Advanced Research in Phenomenology and University Press of America.

Seamon, D. (1984). Phenomenologies of environment and place, *Phenomenology and Pedagogy, 2:* 130–135.

Sinnott, J. (Ed.). *Everyday problem solving: Theory and application* New York: Praeger.

Skeat, W. (1882). *An etymological dictionary of the English language.* Oxford: Clarendon Press.

Staton, J. (1987). The power of responding in dialogue journals. In T. Fulwiler (Ed.), *The journal book* (pp. 47–63). Portsmouth: Boynton/Cook.

Street, A. F. (1992). *Inside nursing: A critical ethnography of clinical nursing practice.* Albany: State University of New York Press.

Travelbee, J. (1966). *Interpersonal aspects of nursing.* Philadelphia: F. A. Davis.

Vandenborn, J. (1982). The proposal as process. In V. Darroch & R. Silvers (Eds.), *Interpretive human studies: An introduction to phenomenological research* (pp. 115–47). Lanham: University Press.

van Manen, M. (1991). *The tact of teaching.* Albany: State University of New York Press.

Younger, J. (1990). Literary works as a mode of knowing. *Image, 22*(1), 39–43.

7

Caring: A Foundation for Becoming Competent

Emily Todd Slunt

Together my students and I wondered: What makes it possible for one to be a nurse? What draws people to want to connect with other people, to be with other people, to help other people? Meaningful relationships, characterized by the exchange of caring, are central to the domain of nursing. In the process of my research I asked, Are meaningful relationships also what guide one towards competence?

The purpose of this research study was to explore the meaning of becoming competent as experienced by nursing students and to make visible the essential nature of the phenomenon of competence in nursing. The lived experience of nursing students in a clinical setting was the source of text to reveal meanings of a student becoming competent as both a learner and nurse.

Working with people is grounded in life histories of nursing students and surfaced through the telling of stories. Students participating in my research study described memorable human interest stories, a calling to people in need and caring relationships. They reflected upon the attraction of an orientation to people in nursing versus the promotion of profit or gain orientation of a business career.

Susan: When I think of business, I think of selling or buying. Nursing, to me, is caring, giving, helping, although maybe it's selling ways of making a better life for people who are ill. Maybe that is a type of sales, but I think it's more a business of caring. (Slunt 1989, p. 85)

As the space between nursing and business was explored, a commonality of selling was discovered. But the types of selling reflected different kinds of relationships. Nursing was seen as selling in the sense of helping another person, whereas a business orientation was perceived as selling to benefit primarily self or the organization. Nursing was recognized as self-rewarding through the enjoyment of caring, helping, and being with people.

Buber (1958) describes relationships as being oriented as "I/It" or "I/Thou," changing at any given point in time. Individuals who relate to things or other persons as objects, through an I/It orientation, use the world to promote personal or organizational projects and endeavors. The I/Thou way of relating is a mutual kind of relationship between self and other. Persons who engage in the realm of I/Thou are responsive and recognize one another as valued and unique human beings capable of engaging in a trusting, open dialogue and shared meanings.

Buber (1965) believes that care is necessary for the I/Thou relationship and that it is in the realm of "between" that care is manifested. Buber describes the creation of a "between" that reduces alienation and allows for authentic human exchange.

The Meaning of Care

To understand the meaning of care, I explored etymological and historical roots as well as descriptions in the literature. The noun *care* is derived from the Old English *caru*, meaning "anxiety, sorrow" (*Webster's* 1975). The Old English verb means "to be troubled, take thought for, have affection or liking for" (Onions 1966). Today we still find the *care* defined as (1) "to take charge of, look after, provide for" but also (2) "to be anxious, solicitous, concerned about" (*Webster's* 1975).

Care in nursing can mean the performance of physical or therapeutic psychological care. Care can also mean the nurse "cares" for a patient in a concerned, thoughtful way. The first meaning reflects the patient as a recipient or object of care, that is, technical care. The second meaning is manifested through a caring relationship between patient and nurse. The meaning of care and caring is derived through context, a particular situation or experience.

As my doctoral study to explore meanings of competence progressed I found that being together in a relationship of care paves the road for the journey toward becoming competent, as understood in the wholeness of the phenomena of competence. "Values of kindliness, concern, caring, and tenderness, generated by art, are buried deep in nursing's consciousness" (Watson 1981, p. 248). As persons venture forth, they journey with caring and nurturing going hand in hand with technical skills and knowledge. The art and science of nursing are intertwined but grounded in the giving of a responsible self.

A Journey toward Becoming Competent

What does it mean to become competent as a nurse? Nursing curricula often overly emphasize the technical, the measurable objectives used to determine students' behavioral changes. However, personal understandings and experiences center on the power of caring in the journey towards competence. Can competence be defined so that both the knowing and caring Being of the nurse are recognized and valued? Can competence be defined so that knowledge is embedded in the continuing call to care?

Professional competence is usually defined as (1) ability adequate for a specific purpose or (2) achievement of specific behaviors and outcomes. As nurses and educators, we are expected to measure performance whether this performance occurs in an examination situation or on the job (D'Costa 1984). Patricia Benner notes the emphasis placed on measuring competence in nursing education and practice. "Carried along by a technological, measurement-oriented age, we have been convinced that many of our problems in nursing education and practice will be solved when we have mastered the current measurement technology available—when we can simply and unequivocally describe the competencies involved in the practice of nursing and measure them" (Benner 1982, p. 303).

I believe that the nature of competence in nursing is considerably more complex than observable, measurable behaviors. Missing in the currently accepted definition is attention to situational demands or context and students' meanings of the nursing experience. A tension is evident between what in a nursing curriculum is typically considered competence by students, faculty, and clinicians and the hidden meanings that possibly exist in nursing practice. The tension led me to begin my search for the meaning of becoming competent by looking to the etymology of *competence.*

Beyond Reduction

The Latin verb *competere* means "to strive together, be fit, suitable" and the participial adjective *competens* builds the definition to include "to be sufficient" and "having ability or capacity" (*Webster's* 1975). In a root sense, then, becoming competent means striving together to be sufficient or adequate and thus gaining a sense of empowerment. The root meaning of *competence* points toward making connections with persons. Aoki (1984) notes that competence as "communal venturing" holds promise for a new awakening of what it means to be competent.

For van Manen, the true significance or meaning of competence is what a person "is"—for a nurse, the very being of nursing. Being can be found in doing. If one fails to turn being into doing, one is absent: "he is not at all" (van Manen 1984b, p. 143). For Heidegger (1962), "being present" was contrasted with remaining distant or aloof, being preoccupied with other thoughts even though physically present.

Van Manen (1984b) furthermore suggests that how one is present to another is more important than what one does. Also, the way someone "is" may influence how actions are understood and interpreted. Competence includes quality or adequacy in the performance of technical skills, but the real meaning lies with the meaning of being while doing. Short (1984) concurs that competence in the form of qualities or state of being is the most comprehensive meaning.

Benner (1985) reminds us that "quality of life can be approached from the perspective of quality of being, and does not need to be approached merely from the perspective of doing and achieving" (p. 5). At critical times a focus on performance assumes priority attention in nursing, and a person is judged competent by an ability to meet a certain expected standard. Nonetheless, the ontological core of nursing competence, the "beingness of nursing" or "being present" with patients, lies within the "doing" of nursing (van Manen 1984b). Being is the grounding for doing. It is through a nurse's knowledge and acts of doing that being is expressed and self is shared with others. The "being present" quality is what allows one to be competent as a nurse and teacher. Do nurses and teachers understand competence as grounded in "being together" or "being present" with persons?

Turning toward Meaning

A research approach to understand meanings called for studying human experience rather than solely giving attention to the outer world of observation. "The rationality concerned with understanding draws its knowledge sources from the interpretive sciences, particularly hermeneutics and phenomenology" (Hultgren 1982, p. 4).

Phenomenology is the study of the life world of persons: "the world as we immediately experience it rather than as we conceptualize, categorize, or theorize about it" (van Manen 1984a, p. 37). Phenomenological studies are context bound and include descriptions of situations rather than preselected variables (Barritt et al. 1979). "Common meanings become apparent when narrative accounts of diverse clinical situations are given with the intentions, context, and meanings intact" (Benner 1984, p. 6). Hermeneutics is the analysis and interpretation of text. This mode of inquiry strives for understanding through reflection, analysis, and interpretation of text. In the process, meanings and underlying intentions of persons in particular situations are revealed.

In my study to understand meanings of experiences within the context of a clinical setting, I spent time with students enrolled in an associate degree nursing education program. (Students who contributed the dialogue in this text are identified by pseudonyms.) The lived experience was that of clinical nursing education in hospital settings. I accompanied students in the clinical setting and became engaged in individual and group dialogue. We also met on campus to further reflect and interpret the nature of experiences. As a researcher, I remained open to new insights as text generation and interpretation proceeded (Slunt 1989).

In committing myself to an interpretive study, I chose to shed the comfort and constraint of the technical paradigm, to remove the subject-object dichotomy and an emphasis on prediction and control—to be free of predefined variables. I stepped into a paradigm that allowed me to venture forth, "making a map of meanings" while putting self into the process of the inquiry (Mooney 1975, p. 184).

> As I looked more deeply with unbounded faith
> I found new meanings to hold and entice me.
> The sense of enclosure is not for one to escape
> Rather the hold allows one to grow, to become, to be.
>
> To grow away from the embrace of surrounding arms
> Is to move both upwards and outward together,
> Coming back again to find comfort and warmth
> Then once again moving beyond but not untethered.
> (Slunt 1989, p. 55)

Phenomenological reflection allowed recurring themes to surface. Students were asked to describe the themes more fully in relationship to becoming competent. Participants were also asked to confirm or redirect my interpretation of themes. Collaborative effort helped to achieve intersubjective agreement, to validate interpretations and lead to deeper understanding.

Tensions in Following the Call

A predominant theme uncovered in the process of interpreting text generated by the group of nursing students was that of tension in following a call to care. It seems as if the notion of caring has been distorted, as students find themselves called upon to be more than caring, nurturing helpers to patients. The National Commission on Nursing Implementation Project and Advertising Council nursing advertisement catches attention with the theme line of "If caring were enough, anyone could be a nurse." In struggling with our image to the public are we not also struggling with a sense of alienation from the very roots of our calling?

Tensions surfaced in the form of contradictions.

1. Nursing is more than caring and nurturance, but, outside the profession, nursing is often not recognized for its rich knowledge base.
2. Caring and nurturance are integral parts of nursing, but the curriculum and hospital setting reward theoretical and performance characteristics.

What a dilemma!

What is the identity of the nursing profession? I ask this knowing that images may constrain, restrict, and distort the meaning of competence (Huebner 1987). Nurses may become subservient to an institution based upon an image of nursing. If nursing is considered a job, then competence is accepted as meeting minimal standards while tolerating frustrations. If nursing is merely technical in its orientation, then equipment operation, skills, and efficiency become the focus for the meaning of competence.

Knowledge and skills alone become a means to an end when nurses lose sight of their calling and submit to those in positions of power. If one becomes competent in responding to the call to care can we assume that competence in both being and doing will be integral to the call? Can nursing be recognized and valued through its emphasis on sustaining the call through both being and doing?

Competent Practice as Integration of Knowledge

I explored what it meant to become competent in an epistemological sense. I found *integration* to be the key word to describe becoming competent in the epistemological realm. As integration of knowledge occurred, intuitive judgments and actions became possible. Intuitive knowing is gradually achieved through integrating knowledge into one's own personal being, personal knowing.

As nurse educators we create structures to organize the vast amount of nursing knowledge and to show the relationship between particulars and the whole of an entity. We give our students something "concrete." Integrating the particulars into a structure or framework is an intermediate process in achieving personal knowing. The structure seems to establish boundaries of expectations and assist a beginning student to approach a patient care situaton. The structure allows a degree of control to engage in decision making and nursing practice. Becky described how she organized an assignment.

Becky: I have my care plan, my assessment paper, my diagnosis book, my drug book, and my own paper so that I can fill in everything from the report and make a schedule for myself. I make sure I include on it everything I have to do from the nurse's chart and the drugs, the nursing Kardex, and new orders so that I don't forget anything. (Slunt 1989, p. 99)

Tracy elaborated upon the helpfulness of structure in the form of objectives:

Tracy: Objectives give you something to keep in mind so when you go into the room you don't look like you don't know what you're doing. You feel more confident about something to say. Something to start with and approach with them. I would feel uncomfortable with myself, I think, if I just walked into the room and started talking to the patient and just stood there and kept going, um, um, and then he or she may think well what does she know? What is she trying to say? (Slunt 1989, p. 99)

Tracy found that the structure of objectives helped her to meet her patient and to bridge the gap in applying the theory to a clinical situation. She acknowledged that she did not feel comfortable with herself. As a novice, she did not yet possess an adequate self-image. She needed concrete structures that, like road maps, could give a sense of direction and ways of proceeding on a journey toward intuitive or personal knowing.

For Polanyi (1969) "personal knowing" means that an external reality can be known through comprehending unspecifiable entities. One acquires knowledge without being aware of its source. Likewise, for Benner and Wrubel (1989), "embodied intelligence" is the capacity to be in a situation in meaningful ways. It is "rapid, unconscious, and nonreflective," a smoothly functioning intelligence (p. 43). Clinical judgments exemplify "personal knowing" or "embodied intelligence," the merging of theory and practice as a way of being.

The concepts of personal knowing and embodied intelligence were alluded to by a student when she talked about the demands of nursing as wanting "to push so much out of you so quickly" (Slunt 1989, p. 101). Nursing knowledge was also described as being "in the back of your head until you need it and it's like, oh, I know that" (Slunt 1989, p. 101). In becoming competent, students begin to recognize an integration of knowing as personal, intuitive, or embodied knowing.

For the beginner, abstract theoretical knowledge allows contextual phenomena to be understood. As competence is gained, theory is integrated into practical knowledge. Connections are made between general knowledge and particular cases.

Practical knowing or doing, "knowing how," is also acquired from practice and experience and leads to clarification, understanding, and the development of theory. Having a context to apply classroom theory or generate personal theory provides the opportunity to integrate knowledge. "When a skill is performed in an actual situation, the characteristics of the situation have as much influence on successful performance as does knowledge of procedural steps for performing the task" (Benner 1982, p. 304). Practice itself is found to be a repository of knowledge: "Students must be immersed in situations that continually call forth the desire for competence; that is, educational situations must be so designed that students acquire knowledge and skills self-organized into systems of increasing power. What has been learned must be repeatedly called forth in situations of greater and more intricate complexity" (Noddings 1984, p. 24).

Affirming knowledge through clinical practice is credited with fostering intuitive judgments. In describing a decision to get her patient out of bed, Tracy stated that being with the patient during the morning helped her to arrive at a decision. Parts or cues seemed to come together to enable pattern recognition leading to judgments.

In looking to gain insight into this judgment through the eyes of the student, I asked Tracy how she would go about teaching a first-year student how to make the decision that a patient could get out of bed. Intuitive knowledge was not recognized by Tracy, although it was evident that intuitive judgments had guided the decision-making process. A rational, rule-driven way of knowing was described. "They could check for their vital signs, color of the skin, taking pulse as patient sits up, noting motor ability, speech and level of consciousness"—all specific assessment skills (Slunt 1989, p. 104).

According to Benner and Tanner (1987), who define intuition as "understanding without a rationale" (p. 23), "the most insightful and significant judgments may be overlooked, devalued, or disbelieved because of an apparent lack of concrete evidence" (p. 29). They believe that intuitive knowledge has not been recognized and rewarded as "legitimate knowledge." I wonder whether the way students achieve foundational knowledge, or the necessity to funnel insights into a structured, objective format for documentation, impedes integration of knowledge and the acknowledgment of intuitive ways of knowing.

Through multiple ways of knowing and the integration of knowledge, competence becomes possible. Seeing a patient with a particular history and illness provides the context and cues. Considering the context or patient cues along with the theory is moving toward competence. The student becomes able to focus on the patient as a person while integrating theoretical and practical knowledge.

Competent Practice as Finding Connectedness

Nursing as a calling is a way of being with people. Included is a seeking to be free from a focus on structure and control and free to realize possibilities and potential in self and others. "Presence, the gift of one's self, cannot be seized or called forth by demand, it can only be given freely and be invoked or evoked" (Paterson & Zderad 1976, p. 17).

Caring sets up the possibility for giving and receiving help (Benner & Wrubel 1989). An oncology nurse expressed this when talking with nursing students: "You give so much and you see it come back. You gain so much when the patient says, 'I'm glad you're my nurse today' or when the family writes back after a death and thanks you for being there and that they miss you. That's what keeps you there" (Slunt 1989, p. 140).

This human dimension of nursing can be found within the technical procedures associated with nursing. Although nurses talk about acts of doing that can be more readily measured and described, it is the weight of caring that is often the dimension that makes a difference. "Presence and the effect of one's presence can be known much more vividly than they can be described" (Paterson & Zderad 1976, p. 14).

Being present and showing love and concern even when cure or restoration to health is no longer possible is a very powerful presence. "It is on this capacity of one human being to receive another human being's expression of feeling and to experience those feelings for oneself that the artistic activity of nursing and caring is based" (Watson 1988, p. 67). In reaching out to another we may ask, What is it like to be a patient and to experience illness? "Even when no treatment is available and no cure is possible, understanding the meaning of the illness for the person and for that person's life is a form of healing, in that such understanding can overcome the sense of alienation, loss of self-understanding, and loss of social integration that accompany illness. (Benner & Wrubel 1989, p. 9)

The art of nursing calls forth intuition in an existential sense. It means knowing oneself and others. A nurse who is in touch with self is more likely to be open with patients. The openness allows one to gain spontaneity and new intuitive insights, that is, "to see what we are not able to describe in words, much less measure" (Eisner 1988, p. 20).

An example of an intuitive insight is knowing what a patient is experiencing within a context of illness. In the following story, Mandy, in addition to knowing the prognosis for her patient was poor, was able to reach beyond the physical manifestations of illness to reach her patient as person. She saw him as a person with real life experiences and feelings. Giving the patient permission to disclose allowed growth for both the patient and the nurse.

Mandy: There is one experience I had with a patient that not only affected me at the time but has left a lasting impression. I was assigned a patient in the IMC [Intermediate Care Unit] with a diagnosis of end-stage COPD [chronic obstructive pulmonary disease] and secondary complication of pneumonia. This was a 74 year old man on a ventilator who was very aware of his condition. He had been hospitalized for several months, and I believe he knew his prognosis was poor. I was assigned to him on the day before Thanksgiving; and, in an attempt to communicate with this man, I remember asking him if he knew what day tomorrow was. He nodded, yes, and clutched my hand. When I further commented that I was sure he had spent many happy Thanksgivings in his life, he began to cry—but then he smiled. I felt in some small way we had established some sense of communication.

Interpretation: Being able to connect with the humanness of the patient beneath all the machines and establishing a sense of communication with this patient had a very profound effect on me. I certainly didn't feel competent caring for the technology that was sustaining this man's life, but I did feel competent that I reached and touched him in some way. (Slunt 1989, p. 117)

Mandy understood the power in the human touch, the power in putting herself in the place of her patient and in anticipating and knowing his unspoken responses during these moments of genuine presence. She did not need a great deal of theoretical knowledge in her background to call up these intuitive insights. They came from within, from her own being or self that she brought to nursing in answering a call to care. In reaching and touching another person, Mandy came to know her own power. She experienced the meaning of a beautiful moment.

As human beings we grow through insights, sharing ourselves with others and learning from others. We find new levels of awareness; that is, we grow and become competent through giving and receiving. Persons have potential for existential knowing, finding insights or new ways of viewing the world, along with epistemological knowing.

Dilemmas Experienced in Being with Patients

The reality of being a nursing student poses dilemmas and the accompanying tension and anxiety may create barriers to finding connectedness. Reaching out to patients in the clinical setting is very different from the focus on technical procedures practiced in a nursing lab. Students frequently lament that situations in the hospital setting are different from those in the campus lab. The critical difference, I believe, is the realness or humanness of the person as patient with feeling; the human dimension within the technical procedures.

Susan: When you read it in a book or you're doing a skill up in the lab on a dummy, you have the basics. You have the knowledge to do that skill. But when you've got a human being laying there who maybe is in pain or who is missing a limb or has decubiti all over and is moaning, it's different. You know, you have the whole person to deal with, and I think in nursing, it's a very heavy load. (Slunt 1989, p. 145)

It's much easier to deal with and talk to a dummy, an inanimate object. People are real persons who have feelings and concerns, can be injured, and misunderstood. What do you say to someone at the end of a lifespan, for example, when uncertainty and increasing physical fraility is what we know to expect? The nursing student may sense a feeling of helplessness when faced with the uncertainty of what to do or say to make things better. Feeling failure to help a person in need may leave one feeling inadequate or vulnerable.

This study revealed a need for students to protect themselves. Inflicting pain or watching a patient suffer is in opposition to the "call to care." "In suffering from something we move inwardly away from it, we establish a distance between our personality and this something" (Frankl 1986, p. 107). Even as a nurse may wear a mask to guard against infectious diseases, so may a nurse or nursing student wear emotional masks. Barriers may be built to protect the self-hood of the nurse. Barriers or protective armor could look like care without caring.

How can we as educators help students to stay openly and authentically with patients? Do we allow students to acknowledge their own vulnerability and limits? Can hurting actually be found to be caring? Can nurses recognize the hurt as caring and not try so hard to shut it out?

The image of a nurse is one who provides all-encompassing care. The student sees self as being in the process of becoming competent and as yet incompetent, another dilemma. An inner awareness that competence is still a goal to be achieved and never an end in itself leaves both student and teacher feeling vulnerable. A nurse is not allowed to be incompetent, and students are concerned that patients may sense their own feelings of incompetence. We hide the "real self" both from our person and others and thus trigger pretending, self-alienation, or behaving as an imposter.

Carol: Sometimes I'll go in there and I'll be fooling with an IV, and the alarm keeps going off and I can't figure it out, and I'll go get the nurse. And here you are trying to act like you know what you're doing. "I know what I'm doing." "Well maybe you better go get the nurse." (Slunt 1989, p. 131)

There is a sense of vulnerability too in being responsible for another person, a real person who can be injured. Students used metaphors related to tasks in other careers to compare the value of a person's life. The comparison was a way to understand the commitment they felt to a real person. For example, a competent auto mechanic can get right to your car and figure out what is wrong and fix it, but the competent nurse has to be able to deal with a human being, not just an arm or leg or whatever. Caring for a real person is not like "selling a hamburger" or "cutting a bolt of fabric." A student compared the stressors that go along with nursing and the lack of stress in working in a fabric store. "In the fabric store if you make a mistake you can just roll up the fabric. You cannot do that with a patient" (Berman with Slunt 1987, p. 8). A person called into nursing is concerned with the value of a life.

Valuing Personhood

Students expressed a valuing of life and personhood in many ways. In the process of becoming competent, they came to know patients in a deeper sense. Experiencing vulnerability may provide the enlightenment to bring persons together, to share the common bond of humanity. Students searched for a better way of Being for those in their care. In extended-care facilities, students searched for hope, peace and happiness in caring for the elderly.

I found Mrs. S. to be a beautiful, well adjusted, kind and tremendously loving and giving individual. As I sat and visited with her, I was incredibly aware of how in the midst of physical suffering and deterioration there are individuals who maintain a spirit, a light, an integrity that transcends their disability. It was a moving and unforgettable experience for me—and it has followed me through other clinical days where the patients were not as psychologically and developmentally at peace with their lives (McCarthy 1990).

With the students, patients often shared their wisdom of life and were cheerleaders for the younger: "I'm proud of you;" "We need you;" "Don't ever give up." In their patients students saw happiness and contentment through a smile, a laugh, and the chance to help others.

Time together, watching, and listening helped students learn how they made a difference. In becoming more aware of self, the power within self may become visible and serve as the source of energy for reaching out to others, for living the call into nursing. More authentic and meaningful encounters become possible. While talking with the person in the story that follows, Tracy communicated by spending time sitting and talking, being genuinely interested and present. I watched as she bent over the patient's very still body, as she wrapped his personal dark blue knit blanket around his shoulders and was touching, stroking, and talking softly. Here is her story about this meaningful experience.

My patient was a no code. He didn't talk to me all morning, but I still continued to communicate to him and talk to him as if he could understand me. Just as I was leaving, he took my hand, opened his eyes, and began speaking clearly to me. He thanked me for caring for him, and also talked about dying. He was 93 years old and was able to tell me that he felt he led a full life and was ready to die. He felt comfortable with death, and this made me also feel comfortable talking with him about it. I also had the opportunity to talk with the family, which was a new experience. I felt I made a difference in this person's life, and it made me feel real good. (Slunt 1989, p. 155)

In writing about a meaningful experience, Tracy reflected upon the meaning of making a difference. Talking with someone, holding a person's hand, and just being with the individual were ways that she used the power of self. The patient responded through being less anxious and more peaceful. An awareness of the emotions of a patient allowed Tracy to value as meaningful the difference her presence made. Tracy, in response, felt closeness and comfort in being with the patient.

The experience of responding to each other was most powerful. Tracy knew she had made a difference and felt competent. She continued to try to understand the powerful force behind the encounter. She shared her experience in a faculty-led conference a few days later, and other students related similar feelings. In turning to the instructor, however, the following dialogue ensued:

Susan: I think we've all had that experience. It's just amazing that the conversation becomes so lucid.

Faculty: It would be one or a combination of physiological possibilities: electrolytes, oxygen, and/or glucose levels.

Val: Could it be psychological?

Faculty: No, I think there would be other cues if it was psychological; other cues of depression would be seen during the morning. I think it's physical. (Slunt 1989, p. 156)

The above dialogue points to the objectivity of the nursing curriculum as patient behavior is interpreted in terms of a disease process. The faculty member felt a need to explain with scientific rationale that which had called the students to wonder and to marvel. It was, however, the unsaid that communicated the art of nursing, the caring, that made a difference.

Although not questioning the faculty member at the time, Tracy later shared that she knew the patient heard her during the morning because he told her things that had happened that morning and thanked her for the care given. "It had to do with just being with him throughout the morning and talking to him the way that I did." Making a difference was possible for Tracy because she was aware of her own personal power. In the process she recognized potential and growth in competence.

New Meanings of Competence

In telling stories of meaningful experiences, themes pointed toward a sense of community. "Together as partners," or "striving together," is also a structure of meaning found in competence. Competence as a nurse means more than restoring health, more than providing therapies. The intersubjective transactional relationships involved in nursing include helping a person "become more" in a particular life situation (Paterson & Zderad 1976, p. 12). In following a call to care for others, in being responsible to others, the nurse may also grow.

Competence is a process of becoming, a process of growth. It evolves, becoming a growing spiral as a person gives of self and receives from others. Self-growth is like a spiral, always tethered to a foundation of Being and moving to and fro. Anxiety and tension as well as plateaus of comfort and a sense of empowerment are found in this evolving process, but the process continues to spiral again and again toward higher levels of competence. The plateaus allow time for reflection and time to be replenished. There seems to be an inner awareness that competence is a goal to be achieved and never an end in itself.

Relating as partners, sharing together, allow one to be and become competent. We invest each other with strength, both comfort and empowerment. The giving of self is balanced by replenishment through receiving from others. How can we help the student see the loving and caring that comes back? When the nursing student is able to make the patient feel better, the nurse also feels better. Patient comfort becomes student comfort.

Meanings of competence include the knowledge and skill for safe and efficient performance, the ongoing quest to understand self and other, and the intertwining of caring with knowing and doing. Completing an assignment, meeting expectations, and providing safe care are ways to be accepted as competent by members of the nursing profession. A meaning of competence is a standard for safe practice.

Understanding self and other is the hope to move away the barriers, the armor, the alienation, the personal suffering; it means to experience an experience and be able to share it. Understanding competence means understanding the call to care as a relationship of knowing, doing, and being. Knowing, doing, and being are interrelated. Being is the beginning, or center, the very essence of personhood. Being present to another is a way of being that reflects caring and concern. One can see the call to care when persons simultaneously engage in activities involving knowing or doing.

Persons unite at the level of Being. A genuine encounter symbolic of mutuality is a union of Beings. A more superficial way of being together is at the knowing and doing levels of interaction. In the process of becoming competent, persons experience an awareness of union with another. A caring way of Being is the foundation for competence as knowing and doing.

Throughout this study I found that competence meant a balance. To balance the technical and human dimensions of nursing, one blends the science and art. In describing competence as being more than skills and knowing that and how, Tracy talked of competence as being the "whole rounded thing" and then added, "in a nutshell." The metaphor was used to put meaning into language. What she could express was so small in comparison to what she was trying to say (Slunt 1989, p. 185).

The difficulty of expressing the "whole rounded" meaning of competence is a phenomenon that frustrates nurses. We often deny our calling both in a practice centered on efficiency and performance and through a curriculum that perpetuates the coldness of facts rather than the warmth associated with individual expression of meaning.

Curriculum for Building Competence upon Caring

What would a nursing curriculum look like that allowed and enabled persons to be touched by human tenderness? Could meeting and caring for others be viewed as an awesome experience full of potential and possibility?

Challenge to Care

One enters a profession such as nursing
Bringing only one's self in answer to a call:
A background rich in experience and deep personal meanings,
But nothing else to hide behind, naked and without walls

Others seem so knowledgeable and efficient
And caring does not seem to open the door.
What matters is not the beacon of light to lead the way
But the need to hide the nakedness of an inner core.

What happens to the real self and the desire?
What happens to the "call to care"?
How can insights and self-awareness come to enlighten?
How can we carry forth, to know, and to dare?

(Slunt 1989, p. 173)

As a nurse educator, I find that students need to reflect upon and converse about the meaning of experiences. Reflection to gain awareness of a situation, along with intuitive knowledge, leads to an understanding of the depth and complexity of nursing. Nurses provide nourishment to another but then need to be replenished by reflecting upon the difference they have made. Reflection contributes to understanding and also leads to action. For students and faculty, questions may surface to heighten new levels of awareness. One may wonder what it is like for a patient to be in a nursing home or what it is like to be fed.

This study also suggests that students use imaging to connect their own past experiences and traditions with those of patients. "Imaging" means entering the realm of the other's experience and possibilities, a "joining of horizons" or finding the "between." In calling forth our images of suffering, despair, and hope, we are able to transcend a view of patients as objects and be more wide-awake to find a person similar to ourselves—to understand a common bond.

The direction of concern is toward the patient as person—that is, it involves looking beyond the patient with a disease that can be approached primarily in a technical mode. To consider illness, we are called to design curriculum to encourage imagination, self-knowledge, and the ability to listen to patients. In this way, "illness can be seen as a way of being in the world as a loss of the familiar that pervades the way things are for someone" (Baron 1985, p. 609). Listening for the inner voice reflects a willingness to learn from others and to let others in—to bring down the walls. Stories allow us to see inside ourselves and others, to hear the inner voice. Stories also allow others to be part of us as they gain new awareness of the inner core or being from which we are with others and experience life. Stories are personal and powerful. They enable a deeper experiencing of competence and a continuous response to the call into nursing.

I suggest that we encourage students to move beyond a focus on skills to engage in dialogue with their patients and to listen for the inner voice. The following story points to a union between nurse and patient through dialogue.

Mandy: I had a patient with multiple sclerosis. I don't know if the pain was so bad, but the uncertainty of her future, and the worry about this exacerbation was particularly bad. I was able to sit with her and discuss it. It helped me and I think her for the moment to just sit and talk a little bit about what she was going through, what she hoped would happen, what she hoped to get out of the hospitalization. She realized she wasn't going to go running any races or anything, but her focus was on being able to care for her family, to go home and to be able to do the housework, not just in a wheelchair. I mean, I know when I left her room I felt better, and I think she seemed more at ease. It wasn't because of any knowledge that I gave her really, because I didn't. It was just one-to-one talking, on a regular person-to-person level! (Slunt 1989, p. 165)

Stories like this one offer us a glimpse of the meaning of illness to the patient and the meaning of the patient's response to the student. Strength evolved for both the nurse and patient when they communicated as equals and with hope. Possibilities were revealed through hope. Hope can serve as a beacon and as a binding force between persons, making them feel less isolated from one another. Through being authentic, persons are comforted and find meaning and possibilities in their lives.

I also suggest that students and faculty stand together rather than standing alone. Conversation for understanding requires being aware of our humanness and meshing as equals rather than through power of one over another. Frankl (1986) refers to "real speaking" as an "act of communion" (p. 243).

Establishing a posture of "being alongside" or "standing with" a student means helping, watching, and supporting rather than "standing over," controlling in a supervisory or hierarchical capacity while providing judgmental statements or "dropping" questions. In a hierarchical relationship, communication flows up one side of the hill and then down another, a barrier impedes. "Being alongside" means sharing the responsibility for student learning. A theme that students repeatedly voice on the journey to become competent is that they feel inadequate in the eyes of the instructor. Students often believe they are not meeting expectations of autonomy and self-sufficiency. Their concern is reflected in comments such as "The look on her face made me feel stupid" or "I feel like she's going to think I'm an idiot" (Slunt 1989, p. 160). How does an instructor live with students so that genuine dialogue is shared? How can dialogue between faculty and students open possibilities for understanding the meaning of supervision? Can faculty listen, raise questions, and enter what is said into a sense of newness or understanding? Called for is mutual respect of personhood without the confinement of social structure and the vulnerability inherent in hierarchical conversations.

I am suggesting what van Manen (1991) calls "tactful speech"; such speech is situation specific and sensitive. Establishing a feeling of connectedness, it is an application of thoughtfulness in action (van Manen 1991).

Tact is what makes the good teacher—the teacher who is in tune with the student and knows when to be upfront and when to hold back in conversation. Tact recognizes the person, senses how a situation is experienced by the other person, and protects what is vulnerable. Tact also heals and enhances self-actualization and growth, strengthening the positive (van Manen 1991). To be tactful together, then, is to comfort and empower, to enhance competence.

Faculty bestowment of trust and affirmation also allows students to be authentic and to feel competent. Likewise, students bestow faculty and staff with authority and respect for their knowledge. A linkage, then, as humans with a common mission is particularly powerful. A partnership is created wherein together the learner and teacher grow, both learning from each other.

How can we make explicit curriculum assumptions as they interface with the personhood of students? Are our curriculum assumptions consistent with what is really helpful for a student becoming competent as a nurse? Can the assumptions be grounded in our own educational experience and be carried forth without truly understanding what our practice means to students?

Called for is an intentional reflective process to examine, interpret, and understand assumptions. "Curriculum building is seen as engagement through the dialogical process by teachers and students" (Berman 1986b, p. 42).

Becoming competent involves striving together, standing alongside, and becoming increasingly more self-confident as a person who is accepted and trusted. In knowing a "person," one can know trust. I am suggesting that we move to build curricula wherein ways of knowing and being present to another are consolidated, that is, ones including curriculum processes that join persons together in dialogue and reflection. In the process of face to face communion, the possibilities of respect and hopefulness give persons the courage and strength to be free, to become competent.

A New Beginning

Becoming a competent nurse is like a circle of seasons. If we enter the circle with spring we think of new life. In the spring we find growth, a spiraling upward and outward, as persons reach new peaks and build stronger foundations. Renewed hope emerges with the blossoming of knowledge and beauty.

The interruption of summer reveals anxiety and tension as growth may struggle to maintain itself especially if a dearth of nourishment or care exists. Summer is also a time to pause and reflect. Hopefully such time replenishes and stimulates new questions preparing the way for fall; a time to return with new determination and new understanding. Metamorphosis begins intertwining the power of art with the wonderment of science.

In coldness of the winter months, the contradictions and tensions of becoming competent may seem overwhelming. One calls upon a rich history of tradition to maintain strength. The tensions are draining but also empowering with the recognition of new possibilities. It is a time to hold on, to maintain a balance, and to prepare for even greater spiraling in the months ahead.

A "seasoned" or competent nurse is able to find hope, to continue to grow amid the anxiety and tension associated with loss, illness, and concern for what may lie ahead. The process of becoming competent evolves, as an upward spiral and is frequently shared with another Being. The movement is nourished and energized through giving and receiving. In the process of becoming competent, persons experience an awareness of union with another. Competence as knowing and doing is possible through a caring way of Being.

Note

1. This work is based on: Slunt 1989.

References

Aoki, T. (1984). Competence in teaching as instrumental and practical action: A critical analysis. In E. Short (Ed.), *Competence: Inquiries into its meaning and acquisition in educational settings* (pp. 71–79). Lanham, MD: University Press of America.

Baron, R. (1985). An introduction to medical phenomenology: I can't hear you while I'm listening. *Annals of Internal Medicine, 103*, 606–10.

Barritt, L., Beekman, A. J., Bleeker, H., & Mulderij, K. (1979). *Meaningful educational research: A descriptive phenomenological approach.* Unpublished manuscript.

Benner, P. (1982). Issues in competency-based testing. *Nursing Outlook, 5*, 303–9.

Benner, P. (1984). *From novice to expert.* Menlo Park, CA: Addison-Wesley.

Benner, P. (1985). Quality of life: A phenomenological perspective on explanation, prediction, and understanding in nursing science. *Advanced Nursing Science, 8*(1), 1–14.

Benner, P., & Tanner, C. (1987). How expert nurses use intuition. *American Journal of Nursing, 87*(1), 23–31.

Benner, P., & Wrubel, J. (1989). *The primacy of caring.* Menlo Park, CA: Addison-Wesley.

Berman, L. M. (1986a, August). Imagining, changing, stablizing: Maintaining momentum. In T. R. Carson (Ed.), *Toward a renaissance of humanity* (pp. 301–12). Bloomington: World Council for Curriculum and Instruction.

Berman, L. M. (1986b). Perception, paradox, and passion: Curriculum for community. *Theory Into Practice, 25*(1), 41–45.

Berman, L. M., with Slunt, E. (1987, April). *Practical dilemmas relative to teaching caring in the clinical setting.* Paper prepared for presentation at the American Educational Research Association Conference, Washington, DC.

Buber, M. (1958). *I and thou* (R. G. Smith, Trans.). New York: Scribner's. (Original work published 1937)

Buber, M. (1965). *Between man and man* (R. G. Smith, Trans.). New York: Macmillan. (Original work published 1947)

D'Costa, A. (1984). *Ensuring job-related validity of nursing licensing examinations.* Monograph Commissioned by National Council of State Boards of Nursing: Chicago.

Eisner, E. (1988). The primacy of experience and the politics of method. *Educational Researcher, 17*(5), 15–20.

Frankl, V. (1986). *The doctor and the soul.* New York: Vintage.

Heidegger, M. (1962). *Being and time.* (J. Macquarrie & E. Robinson, Trans.). New York: Harper & Row. (Original work published 1927)

Huebner, D. (1987). The vocation of teaching. In F. S. Bolin and J. M. Falk (Eds.), *Teacher Renewal: Profesional issues, personal choices* (pp. 17–29). New York: Teachers College Press.

Hultgren, F. (1982). *Reflecting on the meaning of curriculum through a hermeneutic interpretation of student-teaching experience in home economics.* Unpublished doctoral dissertation, Pennsylvania State University, University Park.

McCarthy, S. (1990). Class drafts for NU 101. Nursing Education Program, Howard Community College.

Mooney, R. (1975). The researcher himself. In W. Pinar (Ed.), *Curriculum Theorizing* (pp. 175-207). Berkeley: McCutchan.

Noddings, N. (1984). Competence in teaching: A linguistic analysis. In E. Short (Ed.), *Competence: Inquiries into its meaning and acquisition in educational settings* (pp. 17-28). Lanham, MD: University Press of America.

Onions, C. T. (Ed.). (1966). *The Oxford dictionary of English etymology.* Oxford: Clarendon Press.

Paterson, J., & Zderad, L. (1976). *Humanistic nursing.* New York: John Wiley & Sons.

Polanyi, M. (1969). Knowing and being. In M. Grene (Ed.), *Knowing and being: Essays by Michael Polanyi* (pp. 121-36). Chicago: University of Chicago Press.

Short, E. (1984). Gleanings and possibilities. In E. Short (Ed.), *Competence: Inquiries into its meaning and acquisition in eductional setting* (pp. 161-85). Lanham, MD: University Press of America.

Slunt, E. T. (1989). Becoming competent: A phenomenological inquiry into its meaning by nursing students (Doctoral dissertation, University of Maryland, College Park). *Dissertation Abstracts International, 51,* 1196B.

van Manen, M. (1984a). Practicing phenomenological writing. *Phenomenology + Pedagogy, 2,* 36-69.

van Manen, M. (1984b). Reflections on teacher competence and pedagogic competence. In E. Short (Ed.), *Competence: Inquiries into its meaning and acquisition in educational settings* (pp. 141-58). Lanham, MD: University Press of America.

van Manen, M. (1991). *The tact of teaching.* Albany: State University of New York Press.

Watson, J. (1981). The lost art of nursing. *Nursing Forum, 20,* 244-49.

Watson, J. (1988). *Nursing: Human science and human care.* New York: National League for Nursing.

Webster's new twentieth century dictionary. (1975). Cleveland: Collins + World.

8

A Pedagogy for Caring: Viewing a Student as a Work of Art

Maggie T. Neal

What kind of an experience has the power to so "charm" you and capture your imagination that you feel compelled to write poetry and reflective essays just to survive and understand the events in which you are caught? That is the situation I encountered as a teacher when I became open to the experience of living phenomenologically with students. I found myself being led by the students' dialogue to think about our caring encounters as an experience of "the beautiful." I wondered what it would be like to consider a student, and therefore ultimately myself, as a work of art in creation. This drew me to Gadamer's inquiry of art and aesthetic consciousness and its relationship to caring. I questioned how I might relate to students in such a way that our encounters would allow for a genuine dialogue to lead us back to an "original announcing" of some truths about ourselves and the experience of being teacher and students together.

Some of the experiences of the semester that issued a challenge or "made a claim on us," as Gadamer would prefer to say, are recounted in this chapter. Thus, the process of living in and creating possibilities for authentic caring and a better understanding of our pedagogic encounters is the focus of this chapter.

This inquiry began with a commitment to undergo an experience with a group of nursing students and with a shrouded awareness that the educational theories and the behaviorally orientated curricular models used in nursing were generally inadequate for addressing the complexity of the situations in which I found myself as nurse and teacher. Undergoing an experience with something "means that this something befalls us, strikes us, comes over us, overwhelms and transforms us" (Heidegger 1971, p. 57). Thus, I entered the situation with a commitment to be changed by the process of being open to the "claims" of the pedagogic moments of the semester as I underwent the experience with the students. Questions and conflicts repeatedly arose around what it meant to be involved in a pedagogic relationship and how one was to live humanly in an orientation that tended to emphasize doing over being, to dichotomize thinking and feeling, and to devalue my subjective/intuitive experiences by requiring that attention be given to a more important "objective" reality. The desire to transcend, reconceptualize, or move beyond the bounds of a behaviorally organized curriculum eventually drew me to explore hermeneutic phenomenology and turn away from the cognitive interest I had been pursuing.

As the dialogue with students pointed to the ontological nature of this venture, I used an interpretive framework to give meaning to the pedagogic encounters by uncovering or heightening awareness of the possible meaning structure of the lived experience (Aoki 1985; van Manen 1984). From a research perspective, this inquiry sought to explore phenomenologically the experiences encountered as they presenced themselves. The aim was to grasp the structures of the experiences, their interrelatedness, and how these phenomena came to our awareness.

Over time I began to see how the caring and nurturing presence of nursing was being neglected in education and how that presence could be disclosed more directly through dialogue, reflective writing, and our being together. Of even greater importance, the "claims" made by the experience had the power to reshape the learning experiences and transform our existence. Such hermeneutical understandings, Gadamer suggests, are like unexpected or unplanned events that present us with an overpowering truth (1975, p. 446). Moments of truth that arise from authentic encounters with others. Such truth has a way of opening a place for the secret, for the unthought, for the ineffable (Wield 1986, p. 483). It was to the rich pedagogical experiences that I had passed over—those unexpected and unplanned events that could not be reduced by some conceptual framework—that my attention was drawn.

Openness toward my entering question, *What is it like for nursing students to experience the clinical setting in psychiatric and community health nursing?* quickly revealed the priority of more important questions, including:

1. How do the boundaries of the clinical setting influence learning and the giving of nursing care?
2. What is the nature of dialogue in a clinical setting that supports learning to give care?
3. What kinds of experiences create bonds of caring?

4. How does awareness of family background/experiences allow students to become aware of what they bring to the interpersonal context of nursing practice and the relational bonds they establish with patients in giving nursing care?
5. How does becoming aware of the claims of one's family ties open possibilities for more responsible bonding and caring?
6. How did our being together and the meanings we created influence our development as persons?

The dialogue that is the basis of this inquiry began with an invitation for eight nursing students who were enrolled in the last semester of their baccalaureate program to join me in this venture (Neal 1989).

Developing a Pedagogic Presence

The pedagogic approaches used in the clinical setting tended to be cooperative, and the encounters occurred in a group context. The interpretations and new insights resulting from this inquiry did not come from a cognitive knowing. Rather, they emerged through reflective writing about our experiences, poetry, dialogue, and the telling of our family stories. I defined my relationship with the students as that of "partner;" I stood beside them and we underwent the experiences of the semester and were touched by them. Thus, while the initial reflections and experiences began with individual experiences, the meaning of the experience became manifest in a give-and-take conversation where language was "the medium that joins the I to the Thou and the Thou to the I as a We" (Wright 1986, p. 202). Language as genuine reciprocal conversation makes the joining of *we* possible. This implies understanding through conversation. "It is a living process in which a community of life is lived out" (Gadamer 1975, p. 404). Meaningfulness, then, is based on something prior to language. True understanding is embedded in a fabric of relationships that signify their ontological possibilities as expressed in words and language—the I-Thou structure of a conversation and the speculative structure of language (pp. 221–25, 321–25).

As a way of accounting for the social level of involvement in the learning process, I have chosen to describe several memorable moments that were significant to the group movement. The use of the word *moment* comes from the Latin word *momentum* which is from the verb *movére*. The verb movére (to move) suggests movement and motion. In reference to time, a moment is a short time or a brief space. Moments thus have moving power and are important for understanding and remembering experiences in time. As Verhoeven suggests, a moment becomes a "point of time that serves as a point of departure, impetus to an action, or experience, a transition" (1972, p. 54). Like the experience of encountering a beautiful, fragrant flower, a moment's time soon passes, but the memory of the fragrance lingers on in our experience. These moments, like the appearance of the beautiful, have the character of an event. Events of this nature, like the beautiful, charm us "without being immediately integrated with the whole of our orientation and evaluations" (Gadamer 1975, p. 442). They present "a special task of hermeneutical integration; what is clear is always something surprising as well, like the turning-on of a new light, extending the range of what is to be taken into account" (p. 442).

Pedagogically, it is around these moments that concrete meaning develops and group "history" is shaped. These points are events where momentary circumstances afford an opportunity to discover something and where our heightened awareness allows insights previously hidden to be noticed. They may be moments when a new level of engagement is called for or where discovery leads to introspection. These moments have a way of asserting a truth that "disturbs the horizon that had, until then surrounded us" (Gadamer 1975, p. 442). These points of power and movement are the moments of *Our* experience where new insights and meaning emerge in the dialogical context of *We*.

The Clinical Setting

Psychiatric nursing and community health nursing are quite different from the traditional hospital settings where students spend the majority of their clinical time. Even though most psychiatric settings are located in hospitals, the unit boundaries are radically different from a medical-surgical, pediatric, or intensive care unit. The student must use "self" therapeutically in the absence of all the "technical props" associated with nursing that we have come to depend upon for role identification in most other settings. The student can offer only self directly to another—without hiding behind a lab-coat or uniform, without scissors, without tape, without needles, perhaps even without a nametag or a key to leave the unit. *Beingness*, which is usually secondary to technical *knowingness* in other settings, is the essence of nursing care in a psychiatric setting. Giving psychiatric nursing care is less definable, more boundless, and more open to interpretation. The setting calls for a personal presence and the kind of self-reflection that may set in motion other boundary issues. Where does one find oneself in all this boundary movement? Normal? Abnormal? Sane? Insane? Crazy? Confused?

Similarly, in community health the actual place of practice, the patient's home, is frequently an issue. The student is essentially an invited guest and therefore loses the usual control of the setting experienced in hospital-based nursing. Also, learning about poverty and encountering value differences firsthand entail personal and professional conflicts and struggles. This setting, like psychiatric nursing, has different boundaries. What boundaries are implicit when one is a "guest" in an unfamiliar setting—a home that is very different from your home? Again, where does one find oneself in this situation? Sheltered? Protected? Inexperienced? Losing control, empowered, or both?

What happens to a person when so much seems unfamiliar and at stake? What happens when one's fear of the unknown reveals too much about oneself? How is the "self" made vulnerable by such an experience? The dialogue with students suggests that the personal risks of this course are like those associated with a venture: being in a place that is unfamiliar and where the outcome is not predictable; being engaged in an experience that reveals hidden aspects about oneself; being asked to uncover self-knowledge through reflection; exploring the meanings associated with learning to give nursing care; and meeting a challenge to develop one's potential through a nurturing, caring, concerned, and connected manner of being with persons.[1]

Significant to this venture was the way reflective writing and reciprocal conversation illuminated the experience of learning to give nursing care. Active engagement in the content and the experiences of the course, and the writing and dialoguing about what the experience meant, allowed new realities to be created and discovered as emergent meanings were voiced, often for the first time. Again, we found ourselves understanding *through* language. I found that, while there was much about the process of learning that was shared among the students, the creative process by which each student discovers self, makes meaning, establishes authentic relationships, makes self vulnerable, and learns to care for self and others responsibly is uniquely different. Acknowledging a student's differentness, while sharing what it was possible to become as we worked toward creating a vision of what it was like to give nursing care, had the effect of allowing the centeredness of each individual to emerge more fully.

Moments in the Lived Curriculum

In accepting as a basic ontological view the premise that "being is language," Gadamer (1975) argues that self-presentation is revealed by the hermeneutic experiences of being. Self-presentation leads us to the eventual character of the beautiful and the structures of all understanding (p. 443). Understanding, therefore, "must take place in a linguist form; not that the understanding is subsequently put into words, but in the way in which understanding comes about—whether in the case of a text or a conversation" (p. 341). This notion reflects the unique way that language belongs to the process of understanding (p. 351). Gadamer stresses the importance of language in leading us to the moments, events, or the "thing itself." Then he suggests how, through the "play of language itself," those who understand are drawn into the event where meaning asserts itself (p. 446). Reaching an understanding is more than just self-expression or the assertion of a particular point of view. Understanding, like successful conversation, requires a "transformation into a communion, in which we do not remain what we were" (p. 341). It is a genuine experience in which something asserts itself as truth.

How did the experience put students at risk? What were the possibilities that language brought into play as the students learned to be nurses? As a way of accounting for the experiences and the understandings that resulted, the following moments from the students' psychiatric experience are offered. They represent only a few of the consequential moments that addressed us. One student reflected about the moments we shared: "We have shared moments—moments in which we were one. Moments unique to US—to the 'US' that has grown. From the awkward chatter to the uniting silence. I no longer think alone when we are together, we have come together—for moments. For moments of growth. For moments of weakness grown into strength. Remember now—remember how it was? (Neal 1989, p. 78).

Moments with Psychiatric Patients

As the semester got underway, the students talked about "taking the plunge" as they entered the psychiatric setting. The reality of the clinical setting is not as bad as its anticipation or preconception. Yet, for the new student the process presents many personal challenges and occasional pitfalls, and the setting seems to initially appear as a land of grand illusion. Differentiating between an "objective" reality and a patient's delusional conversation is initially difficult. Discovering that we are all persons who have similar needs and wants is simultaneously comforting and threatening as the stereotypic notions students bring to the setting began to fall away. Personal comfort comes from making it through the first day and from the realization that one is not alone with one's own fear. In fact, the worst fears of this particular group of students' were not realized, even though they first entered the clinical setting on a cold, snowy day, even though the halls had an "icy feeling" and introductions were referred to as "ice breakers."

Preconceived notions about being crazy, being on a locked unit, encountering someone who is hallucinating, and having an expectation that one will meet people who are violent, hostile, aggressive or illogical, has a way of intensifying fear. Even making what would usually be a spontaneous introduction becomes stilted. The following excerpt is from one student's journal about her first day:

> I was worried about how I would start, where I would start, and what I would do. I was standing right inside the door to the ward and Eileen (a staff member) said, "There is Ms. Robinson." I thought "Oh my God—now what?!" I went up and said HELLO. I realized I did the right thing because Ms. Robinson took it from there. Before I knew it, we were chatting like old friends. She told me about her family, her houses, her jobs, etc.—as she saw them.
>
> Later I went to read her chart. I realized that she was not oriented at all. Now I'm back to square one—how do I start? I guess I should be myself (that is being straightforward, factually oriented, and get all the facts). I feel less fearful knowing that. (p. 101)

The students' comments prompted me to ask: What structures define my being? What would enhance my being as I enter this setting? Is this really me or a role that I am being socialized to? What would help a student begin to bond with someone in this setting? I wondered about the invitation I needed to extend to them as they entered this topsy-turvy world.

Other first-day concerns that were uppermost in students' minds centered around being aware of how they asked questions, their body positioning (a "helping" language that seemed to undermine Being present), and use of theory that focused attention on communication skills learned in previous courses (a technical way of being with a patient). Communication skills that I thought had value had become intellectual straightjackets; this is a way that theory "binds" us. Are these skills limitations of our knowledge—or an orientation that once again rivets our attention on *techne* rather than *praxis*, skills rather than conversation, doing rather than being? The following comment made by a student is revealing: "I sat facing a patient, trying to look relaxed, but I knew that I wasn't because when I stood up my back ached." Other students voiced similar concerns. Conspicuous by its absence was the question of how we are called to be present with someone who is experiencing a mental illness. What does it mean to care in this setting? What are the life stories these people have to tell us? What meanings can come from looking at our own tensions and anxiety? Those questions would have to come later, directly from the experience itself. Those would be the questions that would eventually "find us," so to speak.

Later, in reflecting on this experience, one of the students felt that her difficulty on entering stemmed not only from not having a set of protocols to follow but also, even more importantly, from her own expectations of herself. She asked, "What does it mean to be yourself?" "How should I define my role?" "What does planning and giving care require of me?" She said, "I did not feel I had the tools and the background to do this." It was not until later that she could add, "I learned, after practice, what my most effective tool is—myself and my communication."

Upon entering the psychiatric setting, most students were concerned about the potential hostility, violence, or aggression they might encounter. After meeting many patients, students came to realize that these behaviors tended to hold true only for some patients, usually on admission. They quickly became aware of the opposite problem: "how difficult it is to get someone who is quiet to verbalize how they feel" or "to get an apathetic or withdrawn client to do anything at all" or "to help someone feeling doomed or hopeless find a ray of hope."

The difficulties students experienced caused questions to be asked about self. Here is one example: "Is nursing what I really want or a need I'm trying to satisfy in myself? I thought I knew myself—I'm not so sure. Questioning, always questioning. Sometimes answers are hard to find and difficult to face. Sometimes I feel the need to hide from everyone—even myself" (p. 106). Such self-disclosing remarks and questions, which affect the health and well-being of nurses, are often kept "secret" by students and nurses. Larson (1987) calls these troubling thoughts and distressing experiences "helper secrets" that result from feeling inadequate, being angry, being in over one's head, giving that is not reciprocal, facing too many demands, and distancing oneself emotionally and physically from one's work. These are some of the stresses nurses experience when they perceive that they have failed with a patient or when there are discrepancies between the real and the idealized image they hold for themselves as helpers.

Moments in the Group

Even before leaving home, I knew that the day was significant. By the time I arrived at school my neck was stiff. I knew from reading the students' journals that things were tense. This was the day we were scheduled to observe group therapy. While waiting in a small, dark observation room before the patients arrived, the students engaged in a personal and intimate dialogue about the kind of underwear everyone was wearing. I didn't have a clue about how the discussion started. I first thought the content related to anxiety about viewing the intimate details of patients' struggles to get well. There was lots of laughter, spontaneity, silliness, wit, anxiety—and not much control. At one point a student said, "This discussion is inappropriate." Yet the discussion continued. Someone even asked the group therapists' supervisor, who was also observing the group, what kind of shorts he wore. I remember thinking, "Thank goodness Glen has a sense of humor and this is psych!" Where else does such raw emotion present itself?

As soon as we saw the door in the therapy room open we fell silent—"conversation interruptus." The conversation on the other side of the mirror was as revealing and intense as the one I had just witnessed; however, the seriousness of the content and the struggle for insight was dramatically different. The dialogue on the other side of the mirror had a way of putting everyone in touch with their own personal issues. As a student later reflected on the experience she wrote: "I felt drawn to [the] group, as if I were sitting among them. [I] saw many similarities [I] never realized before...They are me in so many ways. These people are all stages of my life. [I] want to attain [the therapist's] position—knowing the right questions to ask, how to reflect and validate my own thoughts, [I] felt exhausted after the meeting, soul searching is hard work (Neal 1989, p. 162).

Toward the end of the group, a student whose father had died at the beginning of the semester left the room. After the session we joined her in the hall. She had become upset when a patient had become tearful. The students and I reconvened in our conference room, and everyone took their turn at sharing their hurt—and everyone seemed to have plenty of it. By the end of the day, I understood what my body had already known that morning. I was really trying to connect in a meaningful way with this group. I had met a great deal of resistance in making the connection. Today it finally happened. The day was both draining and exhilarating. The students' journal entries marked the change.

- I'm tired, my eyes ache. But I am not drained. No instead I feel like a burden has been lifted. To cry like I did this morning felt so good. From time to time I need to cry—cry without ceasing. It's like cleaning my system. (p. 161)
- I can't believe I've made it through these past 2 days. Yesterday was so draining in itself, and then to have to wake up and go to an interview this morning...All of that crying and emotional stuff yesterday must have cleansed my brain and my soul. I did really well on my interview at Shock Trauma today and she offered me the job on the spot. WOW!! How long has it been since I've felt so confident about myself. What a boost!! I knew I had to assert myself and I did. The group has really helped me with that. (p. 161)
- Today was exhausting. It was so weird that one little thing could set us all off. I really felt better though—Knowing that I wasn't the only one who was feeling desperate and at the end of a rope. I really felt good about us as a group. I think that by baring our inner thoughts and feelings, we will be more able to function as a group. It felt good to let it all out!

    I think that's my biggest problem—holding things in, keeping things bottled up. I'm really going to try to work on this—letting people really know how I feel. I've always been a very honest person—Now its time to be honest with myself—let my feelings out. (p. 161)

At that point, I was reminded how phenomenal understanding is different from cognitive knowing. As Gadamer (1975) points out, the hermeneutic experience is a genuine experience where something asserts itself as truth; it is not simply the ordering of knowledge in compartments. I wondered, What had just addressed us as a group?

By reviewing my notes from the preceding week, I tried to understand why grief and loss seemed so prevalent in the group. For some students it was the actual or potential loss of a parent, or being away from family members. For others, it seemed to relate more to factors in their childhood that caused and still were causing pain because of nonresolution. Other issues seemed directly related to course/school work: carelessness, laziness, relationships with faculty, inconsistencies, rigid rules, guilt over having done well by pleasing the teacher, and a concern about leaving the program. One person felt guilty for pursuing her own goals and ignoring the needs of her family members. What were the new possibilities this experience was offering? Where might the expression of vulnerability lead? One student said: "I felt so refreshed after last week—I think we all needed to get the hurt off our chests. I know I did—It's difficult—but it's something I need to do. I feel like the walls that were around each one of us are gone. Now maybe we can step further in our group and use this to our advantage" (Neal 1989, p. 164). Like the students, I was relieved about and felt refreshed by the changes in the group.

After the therapy group observation session, the tone of the students' journals and our conversations were noticeably different. This experience had led to a more self-responsible level of participation. Students began speaking about the great changes—" 'esprit' in the group." Their journal entries and the conversations during the next several weeks reflected the change. Changes the students saw in themselves and future goals were documented in their journals. For example, a student who was struggling to be more open wrote:

I need to extend myself—my secret self—to friends—open the windows. Walls need to come down and let the sun shine in.

Sometimes I feel so afraid—afraid I'll be left alone. I've been hurt so many times before. I'm tired of trying—still holding back—want to let go completely. (Neal 1989, p. 166)

And, a week later she commented:

Friends coming into my secret center—sharing much more open now. Something strange happening to me in group—I feel *very close* to Elizabeth. She is my inner self that I have closed up in my wall—never to be seen again by a stranger—there in lies my shield—love her openness, her honesty with emotions—tears flow, allowing inner hurt out, making room for growth. (p. 166)

Lakoff and Johnson (1980) make the point that "the capacity for self-understanding presupposes the capacity for mutual understanding" (p. 232). We often think that because we have direct access to our own thoughts and feelings and not someone elses, that self-understanding is easy and precedes mutual understanding.

But any really deep understanding of why we do what we do, feel what we feel, change as we change, and even believe what we believe, takes us beyond ourselves. Understanding of ourselves is not unlike other forms of understanding—it comes out of our constant interactions with our physical, cultural, and interpersonal environment...we constantly search out commonalities of experience when we speak with other people, so in self-understanding we are always searching for what unites our own diverse experiences in order to give coherence to our lives. (p. 232)

Students were also making connections by observing others (patients and staff) and gaining insight into their own situation. For example, after observing group therapy and identifying with a patient who was nonassertive, a student further reflected on her own difficulties and linked them directly to her relationship with her mother. She said:

I certainly didn't learn this almost subservient behavior from my mother who is assertive and communicated her feelings very well. It's odd that I haven't initiated this behavior because it is something that I admire her a great deal for. It's possible that I have not been assertive because I have never been able to assert myself with my mother. I always felt that she had too many things to worry about (my parents are divorced) and didn't need to be bothered with things that were bothering me. As I write this I realize that this is silly because what my mother wants is for us to be able to share our feelings. Often I get the feeling she knows things are troubling me, and it probably hurts that I don't share them with her. (Neal 1989, p. 168)

Many of the students were coming to insights that allowed them to see through distortions that had some claim on them. Gadamer (1975) reminds us that "insight is more than knowledge. . . It always involves an escape from something that had deceived us and held us captive" (pp. 319–20).

It was becoming clearer how each student's "caughtness" formed a "conceptual system" that governed much of their everyday functioning with patients and in the group. A conceptual system, says Lakoff and Johnson (1980), is "fundamentally metaphorical in nature" and central in "defining our everyday realities—both thinking and acting" (p. 3). Many of these student issues, while they emerged in the group and in the students' work with patients, seemed even more closely linked to their own personal family stories. Then I noticed how frequently students were writing about their own engagement with their families.

For instance, the student who found it difficult to work with a manipulative patient also wrote about similar issues with her parents and children. She eventually came to see how she played a role in the process and became determined to change her responses in the process. Note the pattern:

Emerging Insight:

> *With parents*—[I] feel I've been triangled all my life with my mom and dad! They won't let go and keep pulling me in. (Neal 1989, p. 169)

> *With patients*—Good week—[I] gained more insight into myself as a person and as a nurse. [I] realize how manipulation works. Big problem area for me—manipulation. How to recognize it and ways to deal with it. [I] realize [I] need to be more skeptical, not so trusting—I accept people and what they say—how can I learn to distinguish when people are playing me? (p. 169)

Emerging Change:

> *With husband and children*—Different feelings are emerging—dealt with honestly, talked openly with my family. I want to remain close to [my children], yet not suffocate them. (p. 169)

Then, the following insight came from doing an ethics paper in a group in another class, a "changing horizon" within self:

Self-understanding:

> I just realized! I cannot even take a stand on an ethics paper because I won't take a definite stand in my life—*No More!* I'm on the move now.

> I worked so hard on [the paper], others didn't. [I] knew a problem existed, but didn't know how to address it. [I] made a choice, the wrong one—no confrontation. My own damn fault—lousy grade. I'm afraid of hurting others, well, what about my feeling? (pp. 169-70)

And later in the semester, she had a chance to test her insight and newfound strength directly in this clinical group.

It was interesting to note how the closeness in the group allowed the metaphors that structured the students' lives to come to life—to come into the open in such a way that the person could accept seeing them. I became aware of how important it was for a student to experience the bounds of a group—a new community, where a different "conversation" would put at risk the "conversation" that had evolved in their families. I believe that it was the experiencing of a new conversational community, in a tradition different from their own, that allowed the insight needed for the students to see their own existential situation and to understand that they had some choice about how they wanted to live their lives. Only then could they also see their own role in the making of their lives. Then, and only then, did they realize that, with changes in themselves, their lives could be otherwise.

The students' journals and our conversations caused me to think about living in a cultural structure that allowed openness and security. How does group closeness permit supportive entry into a maelstrom? How can learning become a place where the hidden is uncovered, where the previously unspoken is said—made deliberately part of our conscious discussion? How do we ask that "gossip," prejudices, and negative qualities be made visible rather than allowed to function behind our backs where they are further denied? Through a caring, negotiated conversation that preserved openness, the experience of this group was rich and concrete enough for the students to learn to live from the tension created by the turbulence and to see possibilities for change. Learning from this kind of immediacy is similar to what Gadamer (1975) refers to as "a connection with the beautiful...the beautiful is a kind of experience that stands out like an enchantment and an adventure within the whole of our experience and presents a special task of hermeneutic integration, what is clear is always something surprising as well, like the turning-on of a new light, extending the range of what is to be taken into account" (p. 442).

It was clear we were in an experience of "the beautiful": we were finally working successfully together, being more honest, being more involved, doing our best, being influenced by truth—allowing truth to have a binding claim on us. Our horizons had been disturbed and a "fusion of horizons" was underway. We were *being together*. We moved on to write and then read our own family stories.

Stories about Families

The family context initially bounds one's emotionality and thus becomes a backdrop for much of our later lived experiences. Our family of origin significantly shapes our fundamental attitudes toward life and provides relational bonds of lasting importance. As such, understanding family ties is the key to understanding the relational bonds we establish with others outside the family and how we experience other groups or settings where boundaries are different from those of our family.

Students were invited to write a narrative story about their family and how their family background contributed to who they were. Later conversations focused on how one's family experience influences who one is, on the relational phenomena established in the group, and on providing nursing care.

Pedagogically, this experience serves several aims. The underlying purpose is to disclose to ourselves just who we are. In order to be effective as a nurse, one must understand and be aware of what one brings to the interpersonal situation. In this exercise the process of reflecting on one's family experience is directed toward allowing the student's relational history to be revealed, felt deeply, and shared with peers through dialogue. How might writing a family story make our being more self-evident to ourselves? How might writing a family story reveal unnoticed patterns about our relational history and the unnoticed barriers they produce? How may storywriting reveal the limits of who I am by exploring the limits of how I understand myself and open up possibilities for who I might become? How can the family experiences of our past speak to us and pose questions in such a way that the meaning is placed in openness? Gadamer (1975) suggests that for real understanding to occur, one must move toward "thinking about that which was unquestionably accepted, and hence not thought about. . .It results from the coming to an end of understanding—a wrong turning at which we get stuck" (p. 337).

Reflecting on past family experiences allows something about the inner essence of the person to be revealed. By looking back and making comparisons, the reconception and redefinition of our family experiences are possible. "The hermeneutic task consists in not covering up this tension by attempting a naive assimilation but consciously bringing it out" (Gadamer 1975, p. 273). This process provides a self-understanding that permits one to more consciously establish "caring" relational values that can be used in giving nursing care.

My interest in having the family theory of the course come to life through the family story did not prepare me for the intensity that was to follow from our writing and then reading to each other the poignant and personal stories we had written. As students began reading their family stories, I was immediately struck by the expressiveness, the concreteness, the authenticity, and the intense energy generated through their self-presentation of the family story. Narrowing their focus to family events, ones that they found important for understanding themselves, intensified the struggles they were most intimately concerned with. A significant event that was a trigger of emotional processes that could activate unresolved issues. Birren (1987) makes a point with which I concur: "Writing an autobiography puts the contradictions, paradoxes and ambivalence of life into perspective. It restores our sense of self-sufficiency and personal identity that has been shaped by the crosscurrents and tides of life" (p. 91).

As the first student read her story, I remembered the many times during the semester that she had written and talked about her desire to become more assertive. There, in her family story, I clearly saw the historic roots of her concern. She wrote,

> It was always stressed that we do the best that we could. My dad is definitely the leader in my family. It has always pretty much been what he says goes. I responded to this by always agreeing and doing whatever I was told, and was very much a "good girl." I lean towards being passive rather than aggressive, much like my mother. (Neal 1989, p. 211)

When the next student read her story, I had a similar experience. I recalled the many times during the semester that she had struggled with herself, her friends and her parents around issues of protectiveness and growing up. She talked about growing up, and her fear that she would cause her mother's chronic illness to become active again. She said,

> I'm not nine years old anymore. But there are times when I feel as scared as that little girl who so desperately wanted to be able to do more for my Mom and Dad. I always tried to do what they wanted me to do because I didn't want Mom to get sick again. (p. 211)

This phenomenon was repeated with the telling of each story. As each story was told, it was apparent how fundamental relational truths about being a member of a family were being disclosed. Relational patterns present in the families suddenly emerged from hiding. The experiences of each person resonated in someone else in the group. Similarities existed between relationships with siblings or parents. Students shared experiences of being hurt by having parents not accept persons they loved. One student wondered what it was like for another student to break out of her "good girl" mold. The comparisons went on and on. I found it interesting that all students expressed problems that were centered in some way with their parents.

Furthermore, the students frequently made connections between the bonding they experienced in their family and their bonding with patients. For example, if they feared rejection from their family, they also feared rejection from patients. If family bonds were perceived to not have been close and nurturing, they wanted patients to also be independent and to do for themselves. If it was difficult to express care in one's family, it was often not shown with patients either. If a student had been nurtured and somewhat protected, that was often the approach used in bonding with a patient. Being called to care seemed to have deep roots growing out of family life.

Some of the same contradictions that surfaced in the student's family were transferred from the family to the patient situation. For example, after writing her family story, one student wondered if her lack of attachment to her parents while growing up made her appear tough; she feared getting hurt from becoming too attached. Did she also limit her involvement with patients as a way to keep herself from being hurt? Similarly, another observed how her close family bonds made her what she was today and, ironically, made her experience a feeling of loss as the patients she cared for made progress. I came to see how closely connected we are to the relational history of our family. "Who we are is through and through historical...It is history that determines our possibilities for understanding ourselves and our world" (Wachterhauser 1986, pp. 7, 9). In other words, the family themes and patterns that are present in us are not accidental; rather, they are essential or ontological: "Who we are is a function of the historical circumstances and community we find ourselves in, the historical language we speak, the historically evolving habits and practices we appropriate, the temporally conditioned problems we take seriously, and the historically conditioned choices we make" (Wachterhauser 1986, p. 7).

I found that reflecting on one's family experiences and interactions has a way of disclosing "being"—bringing forward the being of self-understanding. We told stories to understand better ourselves and our relationships with others. The writing of the family story brought what phenomenologists call a "nonthematic" or "prethematic" awareness of our historical past; this functions as a background for our present experience (Carr 1986; Gadamer 1975).

Furthermore, through reading our family stories we were deeply touched by the lives of others. Through a caring conversation, bonds of friendship and love were developed. We were influenced by truths that were spoken.

How a Call to Nursing Comes to Be

As a way of bringing closure to the semester and the completion of the program, students were asked to write an essay that described how they had come to view nursing. What did it mean for them to be a nurse? What was important to them when giving care to others? They were asked to be descriptive and told that they could write an account of a single experience or a poem or use some other form to present their ideas about nursing.

By that point in the semester, the students had become quite expressive. Yet it took further reading and reflection before I really began to understand how language was being used to give expression to their being: language highlighting the most striking features of the experience; the "casting" of the experiences of the semester in language; language being used to call attention to the meaning of the experience; language creating further meaning through the process of sharing a conversation within a group.

Through the process of writing about their individual experiences, each student brought to the group a different perspective that offered an opportunity for the group to expand its horizon and be enriched by an entirely new and deeper dimension of what it means to be a nurse. Also noteworthy are the unique ways the students wrote about their experiences in nursing, pointing to where *they* and the world meet. Emerging existential questions or issues, while clearly operating as "personal standpoints" or "horizons," we've also shared "signs" possessing the possibility of allowing "a past humanity itself become present to us, in its general relation to the world" (Gadamer 1975, pp. 350, 352).

Several essays described ways in which nursing could make a difference in the experience of illness and in the care patients receive. The desire to make a difference and to bring moments of harmony to the potentially destructive experience of being ill was a theme frequently voiced by students as they wrote of their call to nursing and the desire to care about and be close with patients—nursing is a special way of touching an *other's* life.

A theme often heard from students, the need to defend why they chose nursing, was addressed by three students in this group. They often had to justify their decision to themselves as they pursued a calling in spite of threats to self-esteem from significant others who claimed that they were wasting their intelligence. They frequently heard, "You are so smart, why aren't you going to medical school?" They sometimes begin to wonder why they did choose nursing. Here is one student's reply to her father.

> "I want to be a nurse,"
> I said to my dad.
>
> I didn't really know why,
> but it wasn't a fad.

Well, now I know why
  It's a nurse I want to be
I want to be happy:
  I want to be me.

Nursing is caring,
  and helping along
The road to recovery;
  making sick strong.

To nurse is to treat
  each patient's concern;
To see them as individuals;
  helping them learn.

Nursing is being with people,
  their families, their friends.
Nursing is guiding them through
  the rough—the bends.

"I want to be a Nurse,"
  I said to my dad.
I really know now
  I always had.

Nursing is me;
  It's what I'm about;
It's how I am.
  "I'm a nurse!" I shout.
        (Neal 1989, pp. 123–24)

Even more disturbing than parental/peer questioning of the students' decision to enter nursing were the questions from nurses whose calling had been hushed. Students were sometimes told by nurses in clinical settings that if they were to live their life over again they would not be a nurse. For such persons, one questions if the call to care has lost its meaning. Sometimes students heard, "I would not let my daughter be a nurse." The students often responded with anger, hurt, fear, and confusion. Some asked, What have I gotten myself into? Yet, in spite of encountering very personal questioning of their decision, the need to seek out a challenge, search out meaning, use their intelligence, and gain satisfaction through caring shone through. For students, being called to care had a resounding ring.

Below are two reflective pieces that express the acceptance of a calling—the harmonious and colorful ways that a call is experienced. One can hear the increasingly internal evidence of the students' personal commitment to nursing. As Polanyi (1962) says, "we meet here the powers which call us into being: into our particular form of existence" (p. 321). He believes that the acceptance of a calling evolves from a "deliberate intellectual commitment...These accidents of personal existence [are] the concrete opportunities for exercising our personal responsibility" (p. 322).

This student's reflection on her "calling" has a strong air of commitment about it:

> I don't think that I could have picked a profession in which I could practice my strengths and challenge my weaknesses more. To be able to be myself, be therapeutic and be forced to assert myself. It's a role I can grow into a step at a time with help from my peers, my friends, my family, and my clients. It's a limitless world of opportunities; to care, share, help, and love. A world in which I want to do everything that there is to do. (Neal 1989, p. 127)

Another student piece explores her own calling through verse:

> Reaching, stretching, growing, evolving, caring and changing.
>   Some reasons drew me to a nursing career—
>   Fulfilling needs within myself, I knew not there—
>   Awareness within myself of who I am will draw
>   me closer to you, my friend, my composer,
>   my patient.
> Challenges to continue, to discover, to know and
>   learn.
> Thirsty to drink—taste—savor the flavors
>   of different, yet the same.
> Knowledge exists, skills remain untested
> Time to give, share memories in the still of the night
> Rich with meaning, overflowing in thought
> Sharing sorrows and happiness
> Blue skies and Grey.
> A quiet understanding—thoughts unspoken
>   but understood,
> To move, yet unseen, to channel the energy
>   wrapped in my love for you—my friend.

Beginnings remain purposeful, centered
 on the one,
Masked in uncertainties of accomplishments,
 Shielded from the light, drawn
 and bent,
To stand one day alone, tall, to hear
 the sounds and feel the strokes.
To finally realize, to understand new
 words—nurture, holistic and
 empathy.
Above all, nursing is love
 sharing everything......together. (pp. 128–29)

How does writing contribute to self-understanding? Firstly, sharing these perspectives contributes significantly to our understanding of the call to nursing; they did this by widening our horizon of what it is like for a student to experience the acceptance of a sense of calling. Secondly, and perhaps more importantly, the students' experience in writing shows how the art of writing comes to the aid of thought and understanding. The art of reflective writing is used to help a student "think the material through [by allowing understanding to be] entirely taken up with what is being written about" (Polanyi 1962, p. 355). Thirdly, reading aloud, like participating in a conversation, strengthens the dialectic task of understanding by bringing to life the signs of the text. This awakening calls to our attention a new immediacy about the meanings of the shared text and further strengthens the bonds within the group. Lastly, the tradition of writing and reading about experiences of the semester is a way of making a memory last. On the last clinical day one student reflected, "I think my experience with these people will last a life time." Bleicher (1980) points out that we recognize ourselves as individuals through dialogue with others as we become aware of characteristics in them that we share. Access to another person's life, particularly inner life, comes only by indirect means: "Since inner life is not given in the experiencing of sign, we have to reconstruct it; our lives provide the materials for the completion of the picture of the inner life of Others" (p. 9). The task of understanding, as mediated by language, provides the bridge for bonding with the spiritual self of the other and for "establishing a communion of the human spirit dwelling in all of us and addressing us in multifarious forms from all directions" (p. 9). Understanding of another person's inner life is therefore necessary as well as rewarding.

The Moment to End

As we came to the end of the semester we talked about the places we had been together. As we reminisced about our shared experiences, it was apparent that the moments we shared had transformed our being. One student's journal described the experience this way: "Somewhere in the middle of the semester, probably the day we all cried at the [psychiatric agency], coming and meeting with the group became a pleasure, and not just something I had to do for school" (Neal 1989, pp. 192–93). Other students wrote about how "working in the group had showed them the process of change," how they had "learned to face themselves"—to be authentic persons, how they had "grown from seeing others *face* things," how they had "learned that after pain comes healing," how they were "learning self-discipline" and developing an "internal structure," and how they were "stronger." The following reflection is an example of the recounting of the moments we were placing in our memories:

> In the beginning I thought the purpose of the group would be to work on the project, yes, but I think more importantly, we worked on *ourselves*, as individuals and as a group.
>
> We have all opened ourselves up to each other and I know this may sound corny, but it's beautiful. I can think of no other word to describe it...Each one of us had changed and grown, I can see that. Growing is a painful experience, but its rewards are well worth it. It's funny, but I actually felt myself growing because of the group and the things that we've learned from it.
>
> It's very sad that the end of the group is so close. I will take what I've learned from the group and cherish it forever. More importantly, I'll take what I've learned from the group and *USE* it in other situations and other groups. (p. 194)

Another student wrote about what she had personally gained from the experience.

> I've worked hard and now I've gotten the reward—me—the emerging butterfly. Sometimes it's nice being in a cocoon—warm, secure, shielded from the outside! But [then there is] no room to go beyond the restricted boundary of walled-off feelings. Freedom feels good. (p. 193)

Through the pedagogic moments we shared, new conceptions and ideas about nursing and our life-world unfolded through our conversations. We each had stronger voices that seemed to speak more authentically about our emotions, thoughts, and being. We had become very aware of each other's presence through tears and joy. Through great risks and challenges we had grown older, changed, and become "emotional associates." Through openness and exploration we found new faith in ourselves, nursing, and humanity. By sharing pain, a new understanding about humanity and the humanity associated with being ill developed. A freer energy became available to deepen commitments to nursing, to make oneself vulnerable, and to accept and sustain the call to care.

Encountering the Beautiful

What does it mean to undergo an experience with a group of students? This study began with an invitation for students to join me in a clinical setting in nursing. Along the way, the experience issued many challenges and made many claims on us. I came to see the experience not as a magical adventure to which I could escape but, rather, as an encounter with the beautiful that had the power to make me vulnerable, to transform me, and to make me care more deeply. Was I being approached by a work of art in creation? While the approach was a very human venture, it was not an adventure. There were moral implications and too many risks involved.

A Student as a Work of Art: In Creation

The question that captured my attention was, What would a pedagogy be like if a student were a work of art? To answer the question one would have to begin by considering how a student might resemble a work of art and what could be revealed from such a view. In describing works of art, Gadamer orients us to the following points. A work of art enjoys a unique image that manifests its identity in a unique fashion (1986, pp. 90, 126) and exists in its own right (1975, p. 76). Although a work has a kind of independence, it is still an integral part of "the functional context of life, where it occupies a position of its own" (1986, p. 118). Since a work is unique, but constantly placed in unfamiliar surroundings among other things with their own identity, it acquires a "unity in tension that appears to be organized from within" (p. 90). It possesses a kind of center that supports the self-presentation of its being (p. 43). Gadamer asserts that what distinguishes a work from all other productive achievements of man is its potential to signify "an increase in being" (p. 35). The appearance of the work is always historically bound and temporally situated (pp. 43, 46). The completion of a work derives its measure of completion from its intended purpose and criterion of perfection—a formative process that points beyond and perhaps is never complete in itself (1975, p. 84). He suggests that when something has emerged in such an unrepeatable way it may "be more accurate to call it a creation" (1986, p. 126).

If, for the point of continuing the conversation, we accept that Gadamer's description of what is essential to a work of art could also, in its purest sense, be said about a human being, more particularly a student, what would follow? How would we encounter and "pass judgment" (p. 25) on a student as a work of art in creation? How would we " 'read' the picture" (p. 27) to understand it? How would we judge its "quality or the lack of it" (p. 25) or its beauty or vacuousness (p. 145)? To help answer these above questions, Gadamer orients us to two related concepts.

Gadamer's Concept of "Play"

To be able to pass judgment on a work of art first requires that we identify it, understand it, and allow it to address us. This can only occur if we are genuinely receptive. The "experience of a work can exist only for one who 'plays along,' that is, one who performs in an active way himself" (1986, p. 26). What does it mean to understand in an active way? Gadamer invites us to think about the importance of reading the picture and the use of creative language in understanding the "hermeneutical identity" (p. 26) of the work that is asking to be understood. The work, says Gadamer, "issues a challenge which expects to be met. It requires an answer—an answer that can only be given by someone who accepted the challenge. And the answer must be his own, and given actively. The participant belongs to the play" (p. 26).

Fundamental human play reveals an element of free impulse, repeated movement, and has a form of self-movement. When human play is directed towards reason, our play becomes self-disciplined and we impose an order on our movements "which allows us to set ourselves aims and pursue them consciously, and to outplay this capacity for purposive rationality" (p. 23). Two other points are relevant. Firstly, "no one can avoid playing along with the game" (p. 24). Secondly, being involved has an important communicative aspect in which all participants take part through an inner sharing in the repetitive movement (p. 24).

Genuine communication, in fact, takes place only when the other person shares fully in the understanding of what was imparted—a true showing, as opposed to an appearance, where a false claim or deception is intended to appear to the other (pp. 127–28). "The play of art is a mirror. . .in which we catch sight of ourselves in a way that is often unexpected or unfamiliar: what we are, what we might be, and what we are about" (p. 130).

Entering the experience as a partner clearly placed me in the center of "the play." There were many pictures to be read, not from the outside in, but in terms of the work itself. A work of art is so uniquely integrated that it brings its world with it. My encounters quickly became *our* encounters and their worlds mine as a bonding took place. Gadamer calls this a "fusion of horizons" (1986, p. 273). Some of the truths that made a claim on us related to our own finiteness in the power of fate and to family history in making us who we are. I had to be open to what entered our shared horizon. A significant learning for me centered on how painful and conflictual learning can be. I found that many struggles were so historically rooted in families that, until the students turned and faced their family directly, with insight and self-consciousness, the struggles continued to be present, walled off, never to be intentionally seen again. I found the students' initial self-presentation to be closely related to Gadamer's notion of an "appearance" (1986). An "appearance" he says, is "precisely not an appearance common to both partners, but a deception that is intended to appear simply for the other" (p. 128). This is distinguished from genuine communication, where both partners fully possess knowledge of the whole matter. Encountering others in conversations that are negotiated is therefore important—conversations where more "free play" and self-conscious movement is possible, where one has more room to establish and pursue self-determined goals than one experiences in one's family. This is necessary if one is to "out play" the restrictions of the past that remain present and are being announced through the encounters.

I believe that entering the dialogue as a partner is essential for two reasons. Firstly, it is important to avoid placing oneself in a position of authority or control or establishing oneself as an expert with all the right answers. Both approaches lead to the students' continuing dependency. Secondly, if a teacher is to help students move beyond the bounds or restrictions that come from acquiescing to authority or rebelling against authority in one's family, then clearly another model of social organization that does not reproduce what is familiar is called for. When the teacher enters the group as a partner, it clearly disturbs the expectations that students have about learning. The initial resistance to this unfamiliar experience was strong and consistent. I found myself being tested over and over again around issues of authority and responsibility. However, once a commitment to "the play" was granted, bonding happened quickly. With it came an unmasking that allowed all of us to be more open about our vulnerabilities. I think this process initially only reflected further testing, but at a more personal level. What would this group think of me if I disclosed my pain? How caring would they be? I saw this testing still in the realm of "free play," where conscious choices were made about what was shared. By some tacit agreement, once the group was seen as safe and secure and the bonds as those of caring, the process shifted, the motion in our shared horizon intensified. We became more authentic—more openly vulnerable, critical, angry, caring, and conflictive. A concern related to self-understanding and a desire to understand each person's presence in the group became topical. As tensions and frustration mounted from our encounters with patients and each other, it became even more important to bring those issues into the open. This process was both difficult and initially frightening. We were no longer making "appearances"; a genuine work of art was in creation.

When students were brave enough to uncover or directly show us their "faults," we all learned in the most vivid way. When students moved through "blocks" rather than avoiding them, insight, strength, and self-understanding replaced hesitance, reluctance, and fear. This movement was tension filled. As a teacher, being part of the play and being in the play of the movement called me to be most mindfully and tactfully present as the predetermined structures of the behavioral model fell away. Conversations that helped us understand the movement—what created it and then how to negotiate within it without being done in by it—were what contributed most noticeably to insight and human understanding.

Gadamer's Concept of the Beautiful

Beauty, Gadamer suggests (1986), "defines art as art" (p. 161). Beauty is an invitation to intuition; and that, he says, describes a work. Something beautiful has its own radiance and a vividness that readily suggests its value (p. 162). It is this radiance that keeps us from being seduced by distortions (1975, pp. 434, 438).

Fundamentally, the beautiful "bridges the chasm between the ideal and the real" (1977, p. 15). The beautiful points to human beings' ontological place in the world: through the self-regular movements of the heavens; through opportunities to share in experiences that are unfamiliar in our surroundings; through self-understandings, by which we understand the meaning of an other's experience (pp. 14, 76–7); and through acquisition of "a lasting remembrance of the world" (p. 15). As Gadamer makes a point of telling us, "however unexpected our encounter with beauty may be, it gives us an assurance that the truth does not lie far off and inaccessible to us, but can be encountered in the disorder of reality with all its imperfections, evils, errors, extremes, and fateful confusions" (p. 15). Having the experience of the beautiful "arrests us and compels us to dwell upon the individual appearances itself" (p. 16). The truth we encounter has a binding claim on us and is not simply a subjective expression of taste (p. 18). The experience of the beautiful requires that we be truly present—in complete contact with the whole of the experience (1975, p. 438).

Natural beauty, when directed toward the ideal of a beautiful person whom we encounter, requires that our aesthetic interest also "express a moral dimension, rather than the perfection of the object" (p. 176). This dimension awakens, in the deepest sense, what it means to be human and how humanity encounters itself (1977, p. 167).

The idea of the beautiful moves closer in the direction of the good and is revealed in the search for the good. Gadamer sees this as "its distinguishing mark for the human soul. That which manifests itself in perfect form draws toward it the longing of love" (1975, p. 437). Beauty directly disposes people toward it.

Being in an experience of the beautiful always implies a genuine sharing, a direct connection between the beautiful and our everyday world. This is done through the creation of a community that helps advance a "shared view of the world" (p. 39). This community helps us learn to "read" the picture or script, and it supports our development of a familiar "language of the one who speaks in the creation before us" (p. 39).

Where in this learning experience was beauty most vividly present? What were the encounters of significance that transcended conceptual thought? What challenges or claims did they make on us? I came to see how language was being used to draw us into the play and awaken us to the meaning of the experience in a deeper way.

The Expressive Art of Language

Eventually I questioned further how the art of language could have a significant role in solving the problems of separating who we are from what we do. Students were asked to reflect directly on their experiences in order to understand them more deeply. Asking for an accounting of an experience calls for a viewing of the experience and allows the student to project imaginatively what the experience meant to them. In this study, reflecting on and writing about the experiences most convincingly disclosed what meanings were possible. The writing moved our dialogue beyond the usual case presentations. It filled in the picture and showed us another way to learn to "read" it. Students' initial writing about the unfamiliar clinical world where values were different, where minds were twisted or burned out from drugs, or where someone's world had been turned upside-down by poverty required us to look directly at our commitments and responsibilities to human beings in those situations. Students' narrative writing toward the end of the semester showed what meanings the experiences had for them. If students left unchanged by the experience, then they did not hear the claim that the "art" of nursing was making. As an educator I had to ask, What are those experiences in our immediate situation that allow images of the beautiful to be seen? How might language be used to reawaken or show us the meaning of *being* human in a deeper way?

The Art of Thinking Beautifully

As humans, we live in an interpretive world. That is what makes us uniquely different from other living creatures. This study has not focused on thinking *per se*, even though it began with a cognitive interest. Rather, attention has been drawn to conversations through which a shared understanding was achieved. Gadamer asserts that genuine understanding is a dialectical process that resists reduction. Expanding on this point Ingram (1985) suggests that "true understanding occupies a middle ground which preserves tradition as a vital consequence for the present only by critically excising parochial prejudices and anachronisms" (p. 41). This suggests that a person always resists immediate assimilation of something new into a familiar horizon. Through conversation, the experience of "differentness" challenges one's prejudices and provokes critical reflection. Sometimes sharpening those differences is required for our understanding to change. Uncovering truth and discovering meaning is an infinite process. It involves a process of resistance and change that eventually leads one to a refreshing experience or a new view. Through genuine dialogue, our "parochial horizons are liberated from restrictive prejudices and broadened" (p. 45). Where do we reach our limits of understanding? Where does understanding break down? Where are we when we come to the end of understanding? How does our relational history and implicit memory contribute to this phenomena? How might this knowledge help us understand? How might we become aware of our limits? Not to find the breaking point but rather to see how and where something is limiting—to understand it, to have some choice about it, to be liberated from it, to become stronger.

Through the "we" encounters of the group, the experiences from the lives of others had entered mine. This openness provided me with a new view of pedagogy. Firstly, I came to see how, through reciprocal conversation and a caring structure, the unifying themes of our lives and of nursing could be revealed. Secondly, our understanding of nursing was deepened as we created new meanings in the process. Thinking through the possibilities became a shared experience. The phenomenal path that led to soul searching uncovered rich meaning and much pain. The bonding in the group had a healing power that was energizing and refreshing and moved us through the process. We were each part of the play. We were different historic beings as a result. Our memories captured the understandings and personal changes made through the "spirit" of the group. To undergo an experience is to be transformed by it. I learned that changing one's self-understanding gives rise to new priorities and a vision of new possibilities.

Notes

This chapter is based on "A Room With a View: Uncovering the Essence of the Student Experience in a Clinical Nursing Setting," a doctoral dissertation by Margaret Tetz Neal (1989). A previous draft of this paper received the 1989 Aoki Award for Curriculum Scholarship from *The Journal of Curriculum Theorizing*.

1. For a more detailed discussion of the need to incorporate nurturing capacities and an ethics of care into curricula for women, see Martin's *Reclaiming a Conversation*. She asserts that the goals of education should be nurturing, caring, concern, and connection.

References

Aoki, T. T. (1985). *Toward curriculum inquiry in a new key* (Occasional Paper No. 2, Revised). Edmonton, Alberta: University of Alberta, Department of Secondary Education.

Birren, J. E. (1987). The best of all stories. *Psychology Today, 21*(5), 91–92.

Bleicher, J. (1980). *Contemporary hermeneutics: Hermeneutics as method, philosophy and critique*. New York: Routledge & Kegan Paul.

Carr, D. (1986). *Time, narrative, and history*. Bloomington: Indiana University Press.

Gadamer, H-G. (1976). *Philosophical hermeneutics*. Berkeley: University of California Press.

Gadamer, H-G. (1986). In R. Bernasconi (Ed.), *The relevance of the beautiful and other essays* (N. Walker, Trans.). New York: Cambridge University Press.

Gadamer, H-G. (1975). *Truth and method*. New York: Crossroad.

Heidegger, M. (1971). *On the way to language* (P. Hertz, Trans.). New York: Harper & Row. (Original work published 1959)

Ingram, D. (1985). Hermeneutics and praxis. In R. Hollinger (Ed.), *Hermeneutics and truth* (pp. 32–53). Notre Dame, IN: University of Notre Dame.

Lakoff, G., & Johnson, M. (1980). *Metaphors we live by*. Chicago: University of Chicago Press.

Larson, D. G. (1987). Internal stressors in Nursing: Helper secrets. *Journal of Psychosocial Nursing, 25*(4), 20–27.

Martin, J. R. (1985). *Reclaiming a conversation*. New Haven: Yale University Press.

Neal, M. (1989). A room with a view: Uncovering the essence of the student experience in a clinical nursing setting. *Dissertation Abstracts International, 50*, 2847B (University Microfilms International No. 8924207).

Polanyi, M. (1962). *Personal knowledge: Towards a post-critical philosophy* (corrected ed.) Chicago: University of Chicago Press.

Polanyi, M., & Prosch, H. (1975). *Meaning*. Chicago: University of Chicago Press.

Scudder, J. R., & Mickunas, A. (1985). *Meaning, dialogue, and enculturation: Phenomenological philosophy of education*. Washington, DC: University Press of America.

van Manen, M. (1984). Practicing phenomenological writing. *Phenomenology + Pedagogy, 2*, 36–69.

Verhoeven, C. (1972). *The philosophy of wonder* (M. Foran, Trans.). New York: Macmillan. (Original work published 1967)

Wachterhauser, B. R. (1986). *Hermeneutics and modern philosophy*. Albany: State University of New York Press.

Wiehl, R. (1986). Heidegger, hermeneutics and ontology. In B. R. Wachterhauser (Ed.), *Hermeneutics and modern philosophy* (pp. 460–84). Albany: State University of New York Press.

Wright, K. (1986). Gadamer: The speculative structure of language. In B. R. Wachterhauser (Ed.), *Hermeneutics and modern philosophy* (pp. 193–218). Albany: State University of New York Press.

IV

Sustaining the Call through Being in Possibility

Throughout this text, the reader is called into dialogue and questioning regarding the nature and possibilities of being called to care. This section of the text explores a critical question; that is, how is the call to care sustained? In chapter 9, Louise examines the curriculum challenges necessary to sustain the call to care. She poses the question, If being called to care is central to nursing, what curricular matters need to be highlighted or changed?

In chapter 10, Francine looks reflectively back on the text with a deconstuctive gaze, searching out the tensions and contradictions in the text in an attempt to place more thoughtfully and critically into question what it means to be called to care. In the process, the title of the text itself is called into question as Francine attempts to decenter the "I" in the call to care and refocus on the "caring" itself or on what calls itself "care."

In chapter 11, Mary, Maggie, and Emily address the issue of keeping the call alive through examination of three important themes: listening, being in community, and centering. Mary explores the notion of listening as an ontological commitment that moves beyond the adoption of simple communication techniques and interpersonal dynamics. She contends that in order to perceive a call to care, one must attain this attentive listening presence.

Perceiving the call also necessitates a return to authenticity. A process of centering occurs as persons come to an understanding of who they are in relation to others. Emily explores this notion of centering and its importance for sustaining the call to care.

Listening and centering occur in relation to others. The call to care is lived out in community. Maggie examines the meaning of being in community and explores ways of joining communities through reflection, conversation, and action in order to develop authentic connections among persons with shared interests and concerns.

9

Being Called to Care: Curricular Challenges

Louise M. Berman

In a sense most of this book is a text on curriculum—curriculum from an interpretive perspective. Much of what we have written has as a central concern the meaning of experiences to those undergoing them, the reworking of new experiences which takes into account historical perspectives, the making the strange familiar and the familiar strange. Curriculum from our perspectives offers opportunities for students to share constantly their sense making, their ways of seeing the world. The studies discussed by Emily, Maggie, and Mary give instances of interpretive approaches to curriculum development.

In this chapter the focus is on certain of the commonplaces and challenges of curriculum development within an interpretive orientation. Consideration is briefly given to curricular dilemmas inherent in knowing self, in understanding the milieu, in history and ritual, in teaching knowledge and skills, in moral and ethical reasoning, and in organizational considerations. Finally, attention is given to some ways to get started in curriculum development with an emphasis on being called to care. If being called to care is the central core of nursing, what curricular matters need to be highlighted or changed?

Knowing Self and the Call to Care

Clearly one's insights and experiences influence how one is with another person in a caring relationship. Persons who have not had opportunities to uncover who they are or to find their own voices may not enter into life with others in as rewarding a way as those who through a variety of opportunities have come to know themselves— have come to know what and who calls them to care.

What does knowing self mean? Throughout the text, concepts pertaining to vulnerability, authenticity, and structure have been considered. Starting places in knowing self might provide opportunities for persons to think about the meanings of these terms for themselves. In what situations do individuals feel vulnerable? With whom or in what types of settings do they feel authentic? How does structure support and challenge them? What does structure mean to them? Being called to care means creating ways to cope and deal with the satisfactions and dissatisfactions persons uncover as they plow through the fields of selfhood.

Knowing self also is a frame of mind that allows one's self and others to grow and change. In a sense, aspects of self may be likened to clouds that move and change but are difficult to grasp (Berman 1992). The self's permeability, set of core values, and shifting ways suggest that persons be asked to define themselves not as an end but rather as a process in which they come to know themselves better in different situations or sets of circumstances. The attention to knowing self also suggests that persons take a particularly hard look at themselves during periods of rapid movement or transitions (Schlossberg 1989). Such periods might provide opportunities for persons to consider their initial call to care and the sustaining of the call.

What are some dilemmas in knowing self that persons face as they enter a profession? as they come to a mid-point? as they near retirement? What problems do persons face as they deal with issues of authenticity, structure, and vulnerability? What problems do they face in terms of choice, freedom, and relating to others? These questions are not peculiar to the human service professional. Indeed, libraries and bookstores are ordinarily well stocked with self-help books on matters of improving and changing self. For the human service professional, self-knowledge is a necessity.

The human being is the only being that can transcend itself, that can see possibilities, that is capable of reforming and transforming. Thus, the person has both the opportunity and the responsibility to engage in more self-study in order to relate more richly with others.

Huebner acknowledges the spiritual when he speaks of self-understanding and its relation to forming more rewarding relationships with others.

Every mode of knowing is a mode of being open, vulnerable, and available to the internal and external world. The form of a human being is complete and fixed only at death. Aspects of the self and most of the external world always remain beyond the structures and schemes of knowing. Present forms of knowing are always incomplete, always fallible. Beyond every doubt and certainty is residual doubt. As scientists have pointed out, the only thing known for certain is what is not true, what has been disproved. There is always a better way of being in the world, more complete prediction, more perfect expression of experience and feeling, more just meetings with others. (Huebner 1988, p. 170)

Provision for dialogue with others may take place either in written or in oral form. Invitations to self-disclosure, as well as reading telling works in the humanities provide opportunities for persons to reflect upon themselves, the meaning of the call to care, and their response to the call.

Griffin reminds us that nursing and caring mean the same. Both words are derived from "to nourish" (1983, p. 291). She also says that caring is a primary mode of being in the world (p. 289). The qualities of the nurse then involve being an active participant in the world, having "a mind in possession of its own experience," needing measures of solitude and silence, moving from self-centeredness to awareness of the needs of others, and possessing a good relationship with self in order to sustain relationships with others (pp. 289–95). Griffin asks the question, "How can one take into account the whole person without, in some relevant measure, *being* a whole person?" (p. 292).

Maggie, in her discussion of on the preparation of psychiatric nurses, emphasizes the significance of the moment (chapter 8). May (1991) calls being in the moment "contemplation." Contrary to popular understanding, contemplation does not imply quietness or withdrawal. Instead it is a quality of immediate open presence that is directly involved with "life-as-it-is." (p. 23).

Whether persons gain self-knowledge primarily through reflection in solitude or reflection on "life-as-it-is" being lived will probably depend on the dispositions of the individuals involved. The critical point is that they see self-knowledge as integral to their callings as persons and professionals and have opportunities to gain increasing self-awareness.

Understanding the Milieu and the Call to Care

The preparation of nursing professionals, or for that matter any helping professional, takes place in structures that ordinarily are politically, socially, intellectually, ethically, and economically circumscribed. In other words, the boundaries may be limiting or expansive, depending on the congruity of the preparation of the professional and the milieu in which the individuals practice their professions. At times congruence may exist; more often settings may not enhance the situations in which persons live out their work.

The task, then, is to prepare persons who can sustain their call to care within the milieus in which they find themselves as actors (Fisher & Tronto 1990, p. 39). Thus persons need to relate not only to individuals but also to the larger organizations, bureaucracies, and institutions in which they live and work. The larger issues that may predominate in the collective life may be related to gender, power and conflict, trust, and justice. At times the milieu may seem unfriendly to values inherent in work. Achieving authenticity may be difficult where mutual trust does not exist. One may feel the need always to appear strong rather than vulnerable, if issues pertaining to race and gender have not been resolved within the institution. Structure may be seen as imposed rather than culturally and personally constructed.

What is the meaning of being called to care in settings where persons are seen as objects or as parts to be healed? where reciprocity is nonexistent? where the reward system is inadequate, not valued, or unfair? How can nurses maintain their own self-worth and care for others when the structures within which they work make them unduly vulnerable to pain? How does one maintain authenticity when subtle cues are given that the inauthentic is valued?

Through consideration of real-life contexts, role playing, and simulated situations, persons can deal with the dilemmas in their lives. How can they effectively minister to others? At the same time, how can they bond and band with others to change conditions that are oppressive, unfair or inappropriate? Clearly institutions can be instruments of healing. Finding instances of contexts that encourage the call to care may raise new questions that have not previously been considered. Keeping records of improvements in the workplace may be heartening to all involved. Learning to live in an imperfect world with imperfect structures is important. Learning to join with others in achieving more useful structures is even more critical. Nurses' work has been called both "sacred and profane" (Wolf 1988). The task is one of turning the profane into the sacred, in ameliorating situations that diminish the person and thus lessen the call to care.

History and Ritual

If we accept the assumption that persons make decisions in terms of what makes sense to them, then those individuals who have been the forerunners in any field of study make contributions to their fields in terms of their own times and places. Thus, every field of study changes by virtue of persons who, in being called to care, have seen a gap or knowledge that is no longer pertinent. Such persons have either added to, destroyed, or altered the knowledge of the time.

On this point, Stimpson says:

> education is a series of turns, returns, and detours, not a forced march, not a series of tests, pretests, and measurement of the acquisition of skills. A teacher is neither technocrat, autocrat, nor bureaucrat, but a pilgrim. *Curriculum* is not a fixed, predetermined body of knowledge, but a metaphor. As a metaphor it stands for at least three phenomena: first, the structures within which, through which, and beyond which we recognize each other's being; next the dialogue teachers and students have with each other during the process of education; and finally, an "inheritance," a legacy of human achievement and ruthlessness, the record that one generation passes down to the next for it to play or break. (Stimpson 1991, p. viii)

The task of educators in any field is to know the thinking, theories, and knowledge within their fields of study. Such knowledge, however, needs to be embedded within information about the context and values underlying the inheritance. Then better judgments can be made about what is still appropriate for today and what of the "legacy of human achievement" should be left to the history texts.

Questions such as the following might be considered: How did various practices and knowledge emerge? What contexts called them forth? What in today's contexts might make older theories and practices irrelevant or obsolete? What would be required to create a vision of a preferred future?

Clearly all teaching cannot take into account the historic perspective. Time prohibits such discourse. But as students become immersed in their programs, they might think about what it meant to be called to care in the time that a practice or theory was developed. They might also ask, What in our times or situations calls forth different practices or approaches to the caring arts?

Practices that continue in a precise manner may become ritualized. Rituals growing out of practice may or may not be appropriate from one setting to the next or from one time to the next. What in a setting invites practices to become rituals? What in a particular moment, invites rituals to be reconsidered?

Rituals provide structure and organization within a context and vehicles of mutual understanding within a profession. They can be both sacred and profane. "Day after day nurses participate in the human events of suffering, healing, and dying. Because nurses are intimately involved in these events and because of their caring role, including 'laying on of hands' behaviors, it is not surprising that a system of rituals exists" (Wolf 1988, p. x).

In light of the prominence of rituals, what is the role of ritual in the life of the novice called to care? In the life of the more experienced person? As programs are planned, perhaps attention might be given to providing opportunities for persons to become aware of ritual and its meaning. In some cases persons may set out to change or disrupt ritual that is no longer relevant. In any event, being called to care means dwelling in rites or rituals significant to caring but moving out of rituals that have outlived their usefulness—and knowing when to do which.

Knowledge and Skills and Being Called to Care

Being called to care needs constant nurturing and sustaining, including the teaching of knowledge and skills. Indeed, the call needs to be dynamic, or inappropriate ritualized behavior may ensue. Curricula that focus upon the learning of facts and skills without relating them to the ends for which they are being learned may mean the concealment of the call to care. Those who plan for teaching then live in a tension between planning for students' sharing personal meanings and learning new knowledge and skills.

Street (1992), in her ethnography of nursing, acknowledges the place of technical and practical knowledge in nursing:

Technical knowledge in clinical nursing practice enables nurses to understand and predict the biophysical behavior of their patients and to use this knowledge in the interface with medical technological interventions. An understanding of the causal explanations of biophysical, chemical, psychological, and sensory motor reactions in the systems of the body is essential for the development of skilled nurses able to assess and plan appropriate instrumental action. This use of technical knowledge in nursing has been documented extensively and will not be challenged here. What is being challenged is the totality of a world view in which technical knowledge is *the* normative knowledge by which nursing is constituted and understood. (p. 94)

A major question in nursing or in any of the other helping professions is how to keep the call central when so much knowledge within the profession is considered "technical." Constant attention through seminars, individual conversations, and dialogue journal writing may sustain the call. In addition, a human science context based on "an epistemology that allows not only for empirics but for advancement of esthetics, ethical values, intuition, and process discovery" (Watson 1985, p. 16) is invitational to keeping the call to care alive.

Underpinnings of the arts and ethics allow the call to emerge. For example, in ethics, consideration is frequently given to the meaning of ethical principles or theories for individual cases. In the arts, Beittel with Beittel (1991) discusses the processes of pottery making and talks about persons being *"disciplined toward trained spontaneity"* (p. 122). He compares potting to the work of the professional musician, dancer, athlete, and artist. "A reciprocity is inculcated in which the hand finds form in moving, and the form moves the hand in coming into being" (p. 123). Nursing is an art, as suggested in Maggie's studies. The hand is of utmost importance. Yet it is an extension of that person who is constantly being called to care.

Melosh (1982) indicates the development of a good nurse involves heart, hand, and mind. She writes about the value of "craft skills" in nursing—"gentle hands, a deft injection, careful handling of the patient in pain" (p. 48).

Technical knowledge, aesthetic knowledge, values and ethics, craft knowledge—all are embedded in the call to care. This means that the task in developing the knowledge base for students is not so much to try to separate out the various perspectives on knowledge such as technical, personal, craft, and so forth, nor is it to try to develop grand theories. Rather, the call to educators in the helping professions is to assist students in their own personal sense making or personal theorizing as they learn about and live out their own calls. Noddings (1992) reminds us that in knowing self, others, strangers, ideas, and the world, caring can be an underlying theme.

Moral and Ethical Reasoning and the Call to Care

Being called to care is a profound way of being in the world. It involves intense curiosity about ways of knowing—knowing in a variety of fields and knowing made real and vital. It involves interpersonal relationships based on a thorough knowing of self so that one is confident enough to be able to reach out to others. It involves modes of communicating that take into account both the enhancement of relationship as well as the sharing, building, or transmitting of knowledge. Ethical dimensions are embedded in being called to care. Thus, exquisite judgment is essential as one meets another, frequently at deep levels of pain. Caring ethically is compassion embedded in personal knowing.

Brad Lemley, in describing his sick young son Alex, recounts the care he gives and the care given by nurse Mary. Lemley writes about two ways of showing mercy. He shows his mercy by cuddling his son. Mary cuddles the child on occasion and at other times uses a needle. "My mercy is made only of light; Mary's is made of light and darkness and so it is larger and encloses mine. My mercy makes a small healing, hers makes a bigger one. Alex could live without my cuddling, but not without that needle" (Lemley 1986, p. 27).

Because the judgments of professionals involve darkness and light, and because of their potential to strengthen both those suffering and family and friends of the sufferer, nurses and those in other service professions need much wisdom in knowing how to be with others in ethical ways. Shabatay (1991) writes sensitively about the stranger. Clearly in being with the ill, maimed, or suffering, nurses are relating to persons who may be strange not only to the nurses but to themselves, because of the unusual contexts in which they find themselves or because of their altered personhood. Shabatay (1991) says:

> Whatever the situation, the stranger is one who lives on the edge between her unique world and the world of others she has just entered. The stranger by her presence asks something of us: she asks that her heritage or her condition be respected. This requires that those with whom she comes in contact enter into a dialogical relationship with her. Real dialogue allows for the uniqueness of the other to be brought forth. Such openness to differences is an essential component of caring relationships. (p. 136)

Since health care professionals frequently are dealing with strangers, a curricular challenge is to provide opportunities for students to be able to talk with others appreciatively, regardless of fundamental differences. Elsewhere, Mary has talked about the importance of listening. Here I would like to suggest that speaking so that the other can shed the role of stranger is essential if nurses are living out effectively the call to care.

Noddings (1991) gives help in her consideration of interpersonal reasoning. This manner of speaking involves:

1. an attitude of solicitude and care
2. attention or engrossment
3. flexibility or the ability to shift ends as well as means in conversation
4. effort aimed at cultivating a relationship through building each other's self-esteem and confidence
5. a search through a range of possibilities for an appropriate response to the situation (pp. 157–70)

Noddings suggests that interpersonal reasoning is "moral dialogue among agents who strive to achieve balanced agreement, based on compromises they reach on their joint discovery of interests they hold in common" (p. 158). Nurses and patients ordinarily have things about which to converse. If Noddings's concepts on interpersonal reasoning are to be enacted in nursing, then the attention needs to be given to the manner in which communication is taught as persons gain competence in the knowing, being, and doing of their call.

Moral reasoning may also take place when attention is given to the metaphors that are guiding thinking and behavior. Are the metaphors technical in nature, or are they ones that indicate compassion, heart, and sympathy in living out the call to care? Do metaphors that guide behavior lock persons into compressed spaces, or do they open up thinking and feeling? (Berman 1992; Berman et al. 1991).

Bulger (1982) writes that medicine is now a silent art (p. 2289). Prior to recent scientific advances, medical personnel offered human support. A physical examination may now take place primarily through the use of technology, requiring little interaction between persons and patient. Because treatment of an illness may take place through external tools, persons may lose effectiveness with words. "We are, all too often, uncomfortable with words, embarrassed by them or ineffectual with them, and see them as without value in the fight against a tangible disease. We are more than ever embedded in the silent art" (Bulger 1982, p. 2292). The metaphor Bulger uses to describe human endeavors involving service is that of a "professional sacrament." Webster defines sacrament as "a deeper reality." Thus, if one accepts the above definitions and their interrelation, a human service profession may be seen as a sacrament—a search for a deeper reality. If such a metaphor guided practice, what might be the meaning of the ways we are with persons? of the ways we talk with persons? of curriculum development? of being called to care?

In a similar vein, Fenhagen (1985), in *Invitation to Holiness*, defines "holiness" as the ways we perceive reality and act upon it (p. 10).

"Caring" to Fenhagen is a way of actively using our lives in the service of others (p. ix). He goes on to discuss the quest for wholeness, which involves softening our edges and strengthening our center. Soft edges allow the crossing of boundaries into worlds different from our own. Soft edges also allow creative responses to ideas and situations that might have been threatening (p. 6). If Fenhagen's concepts of holiness and wholeness were to guide curriculum, to guide persons in their searches for better responses to the call to care, what might programs and persons undergoing them be like?

In brief, the search for metaphors to guide thinking and practice allows a creativity and freedom to emerge in our thinking that might not otherwise be there. Freedom is prelude to ethical and moral reasoning, a necessity for those being called to care.

Organizational Considerations in Being Called to Care

The curriculum of any profession invites the establishment of central purposes, priorities, activities, and assessment procedures. Yet have we focused too sharply on the meanings of curriculum to those teaching rather than on the students undergoing it? Have we given enough thought to the patients' meanings of illness? Although the search for more friendly ways of establishing purposes and carrying them out is important, of major significance is the meaning of the curriculum to those undergoing it and to those affected by it.

If being called to care is highlighted in the curriculum, provision may be made for students to keep track of new learning, integration of old learning, eradication of obsolete learning, and the relationship of all of the above to being called to care. One way to accomplish the above is through the use of portfolios, which would accompany students from the beginning of professional study through their careers. Although the responsibility of maintaining the portfolio would be essentially the student's, mentors might assist each student in planning new learning, in thinking about priority areas of concentration the student wishes to develop, and in integrating the new with the old. Through such portfolios, students could keep the call to care dynamic. Students would also have at their disposal tools for reflection as they contemplate next steps. Written text might be accompanied by audiotapes, videotapes, diagrams, letters, journals, and other items that make the professional call come alive. In addition to being useful as the student moves perhaps from an associate or baccalaureate degree to a master's or doctorate, portfolios would be helpful in providing information to potential employers. The development of portfolios in terms of time and mentorships might be considered as curriculum is planned. Making portfolios a vital part of the program may suggest shifts in the way programs are currently organized.

Another organizational consideration is the use of questions in preparation programs. Are students being given answers to questions they have never posed? If students are to engage in inquiry, what priority is given to students' questions? How might students be encouraged to ask increasingly deeper questions? How might students be grouped to find answers to questions common to them? How might journals in which students record questions be used in curriculum development?

In addition, students might be given opportunity for developing inquiry procedures to help them answer their questions. Through an understanding of interpretive inquiry, the analysis of narrative, and the use of ethnographic methods, students can learn to acquire skills central to advancing knowledge within a profession. At the same time they are advancing their own calls to care.

Warming Up: Invitations to Focusing on Being Called to Care

Ted Aoki (1992), in writing about the teacher's responsibility to others, says, "she [the teacher] sees pedagogic teaching not so much as leading that asks followers to follow the leader assuming the leader always knows the way. Rather, she sees it as a responding responsibility to students. Such a leading entails at times a letting go that allows a letting be in students' own becoming" (p. 14). He further discusses the concept that "the curriculum landscape that sustained [curriculum developers] may be slipping into obsolescence" (p. 15). In prescribed curriculum landscapes, students may become "faceless, [but] in the lived curricula, teachers and students are face-to-face" (p. 12).

It is important that curricular experiences seem lively to students involved in them. Teachers, then, need a subtle kind of wisdom. The Chinese characters for a wise leader, or in this case a teacher, would read as follows: "a person who in dwelling with others stands between heaven and earth, listening to the silence, and who upon hearing the word, allows it to speak so others may follow" (Aoki 1992, p. 14).

As soon as existing structures are opened up, questioned, or expanded, persons who are responsible for educating those called to care are called to exercise wisdom. So what might some warming up activities be for those human service educators searching for wisdom and moving toward more face to faceness with students?

Reading

Reading books that may have a fresh twist for one's profession is a way to gain insights that may cause one to amplify, shift, or clarify one's thinking. For example, *On Doctoring* (Reynolds and Stone [1991]) is a collection of stories and poetry on medicine, but many of the insights are drawn from the humanities, and physicians heavily influenced by the humanities. Writers such as Flannery O'Connor, Lewis Thomas, William Carlos Williams, and W. H. Auden are included.

The nature of place is important to the study of any profession. Two thoughtful books are *Space and Place* (Tuan [1977]) and *Curriculum as Social Psychoanalysis: The Significance of Place* (Kincheloe and Pinar [1991]). One can question how place and space influence being called to care.

For thoughtful works on persons, care, and creativity see the works of Martin Buber; *I and Thou* and *Meetings* are useful starting places. Robert Grudin's *The Grace of Great Things: Creativity and Innovation* is a beautiful, thought-provoking work with brief chapters on such human qualities as freedom, self-knowledge, integrity, and imagination. Some persons may find it useful to read works cited elsewhere in this book.

Reflecting on Our Text

Another way to warm up is to reflect on certain of the themes in our text related to the call to care. Consider chapter 1, "What Does It Mean to Be Called to Care?" One might go through each of the concepts in terms of personal meaning.

1. *Finding one's self.* What is the meaning of that term? One can get lost in life. What does such mean? How does one keep from getting lost? What happens when roads diverge?
2. *Seeing the face of the other.* What is the meaning of a face? How does a face invite the call to care?
3. *Entering into.* How do I enter the world—the suffering and pain of the other? What are the paradoxes and contradictions that emerge when I seek to enter the world of the other? How do I avoid Buber's (1973) "mismeetings"? What is the meaning of a person?
4. *Suffering with.* How do I suffer with other persons? What is the meaning of suffering?
5. *Becoming one with.* Can one walk in the shoes of the stranger? What is the meaning of stranger? How does one move from stranger-stranger relationship to person-person relationship? What is the place of caring in this process?

6. *Responding to.* What situations evoke strong responses? How does one learn to let go when a patient needs a different kind of relationship? What does it mean to walk behind?
7. *Hoping with.* How does one hope with a patient in times of crisis? How does hoping with relate to the call to care?
8. *Reflecting upon.* How does one reflect upon the taken for granted in one's field? How does one reconstruct perspectives on a profession within a particular setting?

One might also reflect on the major themes that we have identified as being endemic to the call to care: authenticity, vulnerability, and structure.

1. *Authenticity.* Under what conditions does one feel most authentic? What personal qualities of the other invite authenticity? Sometimes we understand a concept better by considering its opposite. What does inauthenticity mean? What qualities or conditions foster inauthenticity? What in the work place fosters authenticity? inauthenticity?
2. *Structure.* How shall we deal with structure if the stance is taken that the call to care is *not* heightened by replacing one structure with another? If structure is defined as making sense of the world, what is the meaning for persons from structures which have become impermeable? Or where caring is devalued or hidden or invisible?
3. *Vulnerability.* How do persons deal with their vulnerabilities? How do they feel about sharing their vulnerabilities? What in one's own being enables one to feel the pain of the other and yet maintain one's own being able to think and act? How does one become immersed in suffering and yet not drown?
4. *Questioning.* As persons continuously think about being called to care in their own settings, they might think about questions such as those below as well as generate their own questions.

A. What does it mean to be called to care in a variety of contexts—an operating room? a delivery room? with an ill child? with a person with a background different from one's own? in a classroom?
B. How does one inquire into being called to care through interpretive studies? ethnographic studies? historical studies?
C. What is the significance of memory in being called to care? of reminiscence? of story (Lashley 1992)? What called us to care? Is being called to care an event? a way of being? a response to a situation or a person?

D.   How have place and history influenced one's call to care? What in one's background calls the person to care?
E.   What telling pieces of literature have influenced the call to care? What films? tapes? other media?
F.   After viewing a movie such as *The Doctor*, what insights does one get? Or, in a simulated situation, think about how does one in throbbing pain feel while sitting in a hospital waiting room? when one is put through diagnostic tests and waits for results? when one fills out the same form in different parts of a hospital or clinic? when one is placed on a special diet? when one faces several new nurses, doctors, paraprofessionals, chaplains, or social workers over a short period of time? when one is moved from one setting to another? when a roommate is noisy when one is ill? If persons are called to care, how are they with patients in the above situations?
G.   How does being called to care influence how one handles another's anxiety, uncertainty, or physical or emotional pain?
H.   Who or what keeps the call to care ongoing? Where do we get renewed energy to continue caring? What militates against caring? What place does fatigue play in altering the call to care? How might nurse-nurse relationships help sustain and renew the call?
I.   How might side-by-side teaching with professors of nursing and of the arts and humanities bring new insights to being called to care? What common abilities and differences might be found in these two fields of study? In persons who teach them?

Stone (1990) said, "what finally matters is how the human spirit is spent" (p. 351). Being called to care is a process inviting the whole person into the service of others. Curricula focusing on being called to care are characterized by attention to a sense of self; persistent questioning; context, the knowledge appropriate to it, and moral and ethical reasoning; and a deep sense of compassion.

References

Aoki, T. (1992, April). *Legitimating lived curriculum: The other curriculum that teachers in their practical wisdom know.* Paper presented at the Annual Conference of the Association for Supervision and Curriculum Development, New Orleans.

Beittel, K., with Beittel, J. (1991). *A celebration of art and consciousness.* State College, PA: Happy Valley Healing Arts.

Berman, L. M. (1992). My metaphoric journey. *Educational Forum. 56*,(4), 435–41.

Berman, L. M., Hultgren, F. H., Lee, D., Rivkin, M. S., & Roderick, J. A. (1991). *Toward curriculum for being: Voices of educators.* Albany: State University of New York Press.

Buber, M. L. (1958/1973). *I and thou* (2nd ed.). (R. G. Smith, Trans.). New York: Scribner's. (Originally published 1937)

Buber, M. L. (1973). *Meetings.* LaSalle, IL: Open Court.

Bulger, R. (1982). Service as a professional sacrament. *Archives of Internal Medicine 149*, 2289–92.

Fenhagen, J. C. (1985). *Invitation to holiness.* Cambridge: Harper & Row.

Fisher, B., & Tronto, J. (1990). Toward a feminist theory of caring. In E. K. Abel & M. K. Nelson (Eds.), *Circles of care: Work, identity in women's lives* (pp. 35–62). Albany: State University of New York Press.

Griffin, A. P. (1983). A philosophical analysis of caring in nursing. *Journal of Advanced Nursing, 8*, 289–95.

Grudin, R. (1990). *The grace of great things: Creativity and innovation.* New York: Ticknor & Fields.

Huebner, D. E. (1988). Spirituality and knowing. In E. Eisner (Ed.), *Learning and teaching the ways of knowing* Pt 2. (pp. 159–73). Eighty-fourth yearbook of the National Society for the Study of Education. Chicago: University of Chicago Press.

Kincheloe, J. L., & Pinar, W. F. (Ed.). (1991). *Curriculum as social psychoanalysis: The significance of place.* Albany: State University of New York Press.

Lashley, M. (1992). Reminiscence: A biblical basis for telling our stories. *Journal of Christian Nursing, 9.* pp. 4–8.

Lemley, B. (1986, December 14). My baby is very sick. *The Washington Post Magazine*, pp. 26–29.

May, G. (1991). *The awakened heart.* San Francisco: Harper.

Melosh, B. (1982). *The physician's hand.* Philadelphia: Temple University Press.

Merton, R. K., Reader, G., & Kendall, P. L. (Eds.) (1957). *The student-physician.* Cambridge: Harvard University Press.

Noddings, N. (1991). Stories in dialogue: Caring and interpersonal reasoning. In C. Witherell & N. Noddings (Eds.), *Stories lives tell: Narrative and dialogue in education* (pp. 157–70). New York: Teachers College Press.

Noddings, N. (1992). *The challenge to care in schools: An alternative approach to education.* New York: Teachers College Press.

Reynolds, R., & Stone, J. (1991). *On doctoring.* New York: Simon & Schuster.

Schlossberg, N. K. (1989). *Overwhelmed: Coping with life's ups and downs.* Lexington, MA: Lexington Books.

Shabatay, V. (1991). The stranger's story: Who calls and who answers? In C. Witherell & N. Noddings (Eds.) *Stories lives tell: Narrative and dialogue in education* (pp. 136–52). New York: Teachers College Press.

Stimpson, C. R. (1991). Preface. In L. M. Berman, F. H. Hultgren, D. Lee, M. S. Rivkin, & J. Roderick, *Toward Curriculum for being: Voices of educators.* Albany: State University of New York Press.

Stone, J. (1991). Gaudeamus Igitur. In R. Reynolds & J. Stone (Eds.), *On doctoring* (pp. 347–51). New York: Simon & Schuster.

Street, A. F. (1992). *Inside nursing: A critical ethnography of clinical nursing practice.* Albany: State University of New York Press.

Tuan, Y. (1977). *Space and place: The perspective of experience.* Minneapolis: University of Minnesota.

Watson, J. (1985). *Nursing: Human science and human care: A theory of nursing.* Norwalk, CT: Appleton-Century-Crofts.

Wolf, Z. R. (1988). *Nurses' work: The sacred and the profane.* Philadelphia: University of Pennsylvania Press.

10

Being Called to Care—or—Caring Being Called to Be: Do We Have a New Question?

Francine H. Hultgren

> If postmodernism means putting the Word in its place. . .if it means the opening up to critical discourse the lines of enquiry which were formerly prohibited, of evidence which was previously inadmissible so that new and different questions can be asked and new and other voices can begin asking them; if it means the opening up of institutional and discursive spaces within which more fluid and plural social and sexual identities may develop; if it means the erosion of triangular formations of power and knowledge with the expert at the apex and the "masses" at the base, if, in a word, it enhances our collective (and democratic) sense of possibility, then I for one am a postmodernist.
>
> Dick Hebdige, *Hiding in the Light*

While the purpose of this chapter is not to convince one to become a postmodernist, it is an attempt to try and do what Hebdige (1989), along with Giroux (1991), acknowledge as the two most important contributions of postmodern thinking in relation to the notion of questioning: opening up discourse spaces and disrupting power relations. In this chapter I look back on the text with a deconstructive gaze to place it into turbulence. This gaze helps us reflect more thoughtfully and critically on the question of what it means to be called to care. The intent, then, is not to search for a hidden unity in the text but maybe rather to locate disunity by searching out the tensions, oppositions, and possibly incoherence. In the process there is an attempt to make our now familiar text somewhat strange so as not to become overly engrossed in our circle of subjective understanding— refusing to privilege the Being of ourselves.

As a starting point, the title of the book itself will be called into question and turned upside down in order to seek a decentering of the "I" presupposed in "Being Called to Care." To place *"caring* being called," rather the *"our* being called," at the center of our attention opens up the opportunity to look at the calling that is caring more deeply and to question once again what is excluded by what calls itself care. By inverting the focus in this way we might address Gadamer's (1975) philosophic concern: What happens over and above our wanting and doing? In the process we disrupt our focus on self and the tension between technological knowing and Being. Instead we look at what makes it possible for caring being called to "Be."

If we wonder about the origin of what calls for a response in relation to caring, Rilke's words (quoted in Gadamer 1975) are instructive here:

> Catch only what you've thrown yourself, all is
> mere skill and little gain;
> but when you're suddenly the catcher of a ball
> thrown by an eternal partner
> with accurate and measured swing
> towards you, to your centre, in an arch
> from the great bridgebuilding of God;
> why catching then becomes a power—
> not yours, a world's. (p. v)

If the vulnerability of the face (the eternal partner in the call) summons the call to care, how might we be more attentive to this call that is caring and return the power of caring to the caller and not to the called? What is the difference that confronts us here? If we insert *ourselves* rather than the other at the center of the call, do we lose sight and sound of the caller and focus too narrowly on what we *do* in the call *to care,* even though it is couched in terms of Being rather than doing? Have we not yet broken out of the confining structure that looks for the "how"? As much as our language has taken an interpretive turn, have we not become vulnerable enough to admit that caring cannot be possessed in a way that we possess a skill? Caring is something that we must continually redeem, retrieve, regain, and recapture each time we are called to be in caring encounters. If we were to return to the more primordial aspects of a calling as Maggie suggests, what might we find that lurks concealed? What is the place to where we are recalled in our recovery of caring? Might it be a place where we are involved through our bodies as well as our selves? And what different kinds of body involvement might we find? Bottorff (1991) says:

The act of the skillful hand is a depersonalized act...The hand that offers possibilities for comfort is a knowing hand of a different kind. This hand does not touch a body of blood vessels, muscles, nerve and bones, but rather it touches the body of a living person...This caring hand...is guided by a knowledge of a sensitive kind, a knowledge that has as its end thoughtful, caring action...a direct contact between two human beings. Perhaps it is only a caring hand that comforts. (p. 247)

Tales, stories, fictions, autobiographies allow us to keep in sight and hearing our bodies as well as our selves. Telling, writing, reading, and listening to life stories (one's own and others) allows for a primal discovery of an embodied knowing and the power and integrity of the other. But, as Grumet (1990) says:

If telling a story requires giving oneself away, then we are obligated to devise a method of receiving stories that mediates the space between the self that tells, the self that told, and the self that listens: a method that returns a story to the teller that is both hers and not hers, that contains herself in good company. (p. 70)

The following story and response were written by two graduate students in a phenomenological writing class[1] to help surface questions about the way one is called to be with others through an autobiographical sketch or story. The story ("Robbie's Story"), written by Roberta Walsh, offers us a look at the meaning of being called to nursing, and the response ("Robbie's Song"), written by Jim Carpenter, offers an example of a way of giving back the story to the teller patterned after the Reply form of Reason and Hawkins (1988).

Robbie's Story

By Roberta Walsh

My story begins in the foothills of the Pocono Mountains in Pennsylvania. I was the first-born of three children in a very Irish-Catholic family. My father worked for the newspaper, my mother was (and still is and always will be) a registered nurse. I remember always being very proud to say that she was a nurse. She was impressive in her gentle but commanding control in the usual childhood emergencies in the neighborhood. The neighbors often came to our house for her advice or ministrations which she generously gave. People ask me if that's why I became a nurse.

I have to answer honestly that I don't think so. I never wanted to be a nurse when I was a child. I can't recall ever playing nurse. Having spent all of my elementary and high school years in Catholic schools taught by nuns, I always believed that I would receive word of my vocation from God. Looking back now, I think that I must have thought that one's calling came like a phone call from heaven. The phone would ring, God would say: "Robbie, you are called to be a nurse. Good-bye and good luck," and that would be that. But the phone call never came.

I was in high school during the late 60s and, young as I was, I was greatly influenced by the message of love and peace and brotherhood that I heard in the music. I still believe in that message. It's the message I try to live through nursing.

I went to a small Catholic women's college and studied writing but after a year and a half of that I yearned to be doing something to help my fellow human beings. This is when I decided to be a nurse. The decision seems to have come out of the blue. Maybe that was my phone call after all.

While in nursing school, I worked as a nurses' aide at a nursing home, a job I loved. This is where I found myself. I was good for the elderly residents; they were good for me. I knew that my life was meant for this and that someday I would come back to it. But first, after nursing school, I needed to get that all-important EXPERIENCE. The old-timer nurses said: "Get your med-surg experience, then you can work anywhere."

I heeded their advice and spent several miserable years working med-surg units in various hospitals. Working short, working over-time, passing pills, soothing physicians' egos, doing mountains of paperwork, running halls, answering phones, never having enough time to talk with my patients, never having time to nurse my patients. I remember some of their faces to this day, eyes filled with pain and fear reaching out to me for hope, for comfort, and how I failed them because I didn't have enough time.

I learned a lot from this EXPERIENCE. I learned that nursing had to change. I learned that it had to change from the top because nobody was listening to us at the bottom. So I returned to school. And to nursing in the nursing home. Here I had more time, not always enough, but more, to know my patients. I became a clinical specialist in gerontological nursing. I taught community health nursing for a while and loved this too; most of our clients were elderly. I started a family support group for relatives of nursing home residents and facilitated it for six years. But there were still

problems that I saw that I couldn't change. I needed to know more,
I needed more skills, I needed to get people to listen to me.

So that's how I ended up here in the nursing doctoral
program at Maryland. I am learning the research skills that I need
to be able to make a change in the way we care for the elderly
in our nursing homes and in our communities. I also want to help
change the way we treat the nurses' aides who give most of the
physical care to our dependent elderly. You could say that I have
a vested interest in them.

I know that the positivist quantitative approach can't answer
all my questions and sometimes it scares me. One evening last
fall, as I read study after study on the elderly I suddenly realized
that I was becoming immune to numbers. I was losing sight of
the people those numbers stood for; they were lost. I was very
frightened by this realization. I am in this course because I have
to learn how to know the people behind the numbers.

In response to Robbie's Story, Jim Carpenter offers the following
reply, an expressive way to give shape to the feelings and ideas arising
from the story. Jim returns the story to Robbie in a telling that is both
hers and not hers, one that allows for a new listening and, possibly,
another new telling.

Robbie's Song

by Jim Carpenter

Father spread the news; Mother was a nurse.
Robbie spreads the news; Mother is a nurse.
Neighbors spread the news: Robbie's mother is a nurse.
  see the people come. . .the harried mothers pulling
  children with stings of bees and de-skinned knees,
  and seas of tears and seas of fears hush,
  and tears hush, mother hears hush sh,
  fears cease, and seas cease, sh
  and Robbie sees the ceasing,
  and Robbie hears the hushing
                    for
She has a calling.
She cannot lose.
She only has to find the clues, and
Hear the calling of the. . .
  Muse. . .ick. . .music, Music, MUSIC
  Magic Music All You Really Need Is Love, ya ta da ta da,

Just Give Peace a Chance as you wait by the phone Lean On Me
Brother cause I'll Be There Is A season, So Turn when
the phone rings Oh, Let It Please Be Him. . .
Hello, God?. . .Yes! You want me to be a What? Oh, give me a
clue. A writer? Did you say a writer?
I think that's it. Yes. A messenger.
No!
To write, to be, YES!
or not to be, No!
a writer, to write what, for whom, about what, for what for, about
   what,
people,
what for about people, what about people. . .what about People!
WHAT ABOUT PEOPLE? Yeeeeeessssss!
YES!

FLASH! MESSAGE FOR ROBBIE!
BE A NURSE!

she's happy now for now she can say. . .
I got the message; I'm meant to be a nurse.
I heard the message; I want to be a nurse.
I heed the message; now how can I be a nurse?
Give me more messages, give me more news,
Give me more music, send me more clues,
Learning to be a nurse is what I choose.
Learning to be, let's see, A part time job with the elderly, need to
aid, a need to learn to be
A nurse, to be a nurse's aid, to be too elderly, to be a home,
Let's see to aid the elderly, a home, a nurse!
I See! I Know! I Hear!
I have to go; I'll be back—I Know! I Promise!
I love you!
SOROBBIEHEEDEDTHEVOICEOFTHEWISEOLDCRONIES
   ANDWENTINTOAPLACEMUCHLIKEPURGATORY
the mundane, piles of paper,
piles of patients, pain,
pampering pediatricians, pushing pills, perceiving
pain, patients piercing pain,
pausing for patients, NO, please,
pain in patients eyes, please,
perceiving pleas,
NO, push papers, piles of pills, piles of pleas, please, their eyes,

pain in patients eyes, listen,
and pleas and cries and piercing sighs,
hear,
please let me
pause and
ease the sighs, and hush the cries and cease the seas,
PLEASE hear my pleas and
pause
and LET ME pause
and hear. . .
    my heart, pause
and let me hear my heart, their hearts, pause/
   break
my heart's plea,
   please
     pause. . .
   I must move on
   for
   I have a song to sing!
see the people come. . .the harried children pulling
mothers and fathers with aching hearts and failing knees,
and seas of tears and seas of fears hush.
and tears hush, someone hears hush sh
fears ease, and seas cease, sh
for Robbie sees to the ceasing,
and Robbie hears the hushing
   sing the good news!
   SING THE GOOD NEWS!

The power in the story and the reply illustrate the embodied sense of the call as experienced through the sight and sounds of those calling. Caring is called to "be" through an announcing of the caring being Robbie has always been. In relation to the book and its focus on "Being Called to Care," we now might ask: Beyond Being—Where To? Who is the caller and who is the called? What is being called in the call?

Conscience as the Call of Care: A Retrieval of Self through the Other

The theme of authenticity is a direct link to the question of Where to? in the movement "beyond Being." While I have suggested that we might refocus our attention on *caring* being called rather *our* being called to care, Heidegger (1962) reminds us that self gets brought back to itself through conscience as it manifests itself as the call of care. The caller is self (being anxious about its potentiality for Being) as well as the called (being summoned back from being given over to the "they"). It is a lostness in the "they" (tasks, rules, standards, and urgencies of the world) already decided upon that keep the self from taking hold of its possibilities of Being, and as it gets carried along, ensnares itself in inauthenticity. "The appeal to the they-self signifies summoning one's ownmost Self to its potentiality-for-Being. . .that is, as concernful Being-in-the-world and Being with Others" (Heidegger 1962, p. 325). He is suggesting, then, that the call comes from self and yet beyond self and over self. In order to allow these dimensions of calling, one has to become free for the call, that is, have a readiness for the potentiality of getting appealed to or having a claim made upon oneself.

In an analysis of understanding a patient's fear of gold shots in the treatment of rheumatoid arthritis, Hovanec (1982) illustrates her going beyond herself and beyond what was said to her in the appeal made by the patient. It was a confounding experience to Hovanec because of her wanting to implement a comfort measure for the fear rather than staying with the patient's feelings of being frightened. What Hovanec also acknowledged confronting was her own feeling of anger and helplessness to do anything about the rheumatoid arthritis that had invaded this woman's body. If she had been able to stay with the patient's words and recognize her own sense of bewilderment and surprise at being rendered helpless, she might have been able to evolve her surprise to a curiosity about the fear dimension and thus understand it better. She began to sense that she was focusing more on withholding information than seeking more information from the patient about her fears. The other's fear and pain became as much a struggle with self as with the Other, and thus prevented her from really being receptive to the call. Her identity as nurse and its demands exploded in her relation with the Other—the patient.

This example might also illustrate what the book's other two themes of vulnerability and structure give rise to. Changing the structure of care from an immediate problem solving response to reduce fear and pain (Doing), to a feeling-staying response (Being), creates an opportunity to experience the vulnerability faced through uncertainty and the breaking out from learned structures which tend to work against Being. This hermeneutic response savors ambiguity and is willing to face the difficulty it evokes without withdrawing. It also illustrates the dialectic tension between the reality of how care in nursing practice has been socially formed and the possibility for what it could become.

Mary speaks about needing to nurture a new language of lived vulnerability, and Maggie asks, What would a structure look like that encourages vulnerability? Emily calls for a new structure that might allow for greater authenticity of the person. What is it that these concerns are really questioning in relation to care? Rather than questioning the meaning of being called to care are we being questioned by care itself?—and thus again the emergence of a new question in relation to *caring* being called rather than *our* being called? What is it about care and its structure and language that has not yet been articulated? What kind of "abnormal discourse" might bring us to entering "spaces of nakedness" that Mary suggests might prove fruitful? How is our present language placed into turbulence by such questions? If hermeneutic interpretation is a recovery of a prior understanding for which we have lacked words, what is it that might be recovered from disrupting the binary opposition of Doing/Being in order to hear what is calling in the call?

When the call is understood with an existential kind of hearing, we might find a new direction and language of vulnerability in Heidegger's (1962) claim that "Being-guilty constitutes the Being to which we give the name of care" (p. 332–33). Being-guilty has the signification of being responsible for, and in the idea of guilty there lies the character of a "not." Guilty is seen as being the basis for a being which has been defined by a "not." As we have struggled with trying to break away from technological determination, have we in this sense been struggling with our own inauthenticity, of being determined by a "not," an absence, a "not" Being? Are we seeking to assume responsibility for our lostness in the "they" and thus Being-guilty for it? Has the call to care been a summons to Being-guilty in this sense? If indeed the call to care gives us a sense of Being-guilty, this calling back is a calling forth of our potentiality for being the caring beings we have always been. Now we might be led to ask: How can we speak of caring from this place of Being-guilty? and What is the ontological source of "not-ness" that the Other helps to recall?

Note

1. Appreciation is given to Robbie Walsh and Jim Carpenter for consenting to share their sensitively rendered narratives written in a graduate course I taught at the University of Maryland, summer 1992. Roberta is a clinical specialist in gerontological nursing, and Jim is a high school drama teacher.

References

Bottorff, J. (1991). The lived experience of being comforted by a nurse. *Phenomenology + Pedagogy, 9*, 237–52.

Gadamer, H. G. (1975). *Truth and method*. New York: Crossroad.

Giroux, H. A. (Ed.). (1991). *Postmodernism, feminism, and cultural politics: Redrawing educational boundaries*. Albany: State University of New York Press.

Grumet, M. (1990). The politics of personal knowledge. In C. Witherell & N. Noddings (Eds.), *Stories lives tell: Narrative and dialogue in education* (pp. 67–77). New York: Teachers College Press.

Hebdige, D. (1989). *Hiding in the light*. New York: Routledge.

Heidegger, M. (1962). *Being and time* (J. Macquarrie & E. Robinson, Trans.). New York: Harper & Row. (Original work published 1927)

Hovanec, M. (1982). A transformation of understanding. In V. Darroch & R. Silvers (Eds.), *Interpretive human studies: An introduction to phenomenological research* (pp. 165–72). Washington, D.C.: University Press of America.

Reason, P., & Hawkins, P. (1988). Storytelling as inquiry. In P. Reason (Ed.), *Human inquiry in action: Developments in new paradigm research* (pp. 79–101). Beverly Hills: Sage Publications.

Keeping the Call Alive

Mary Ellen Lashley, Maggie T. Neal, and Emily Todd Slunt

Responding to the call to care may be a one-time act or a sustained life commitment. Throughout this text, we have explored what it means to be called to care. We have inquired into ways of responding to the call and explored contexts in which the call to care is experienced.

In this chapter, we address the question, What sustains the call to care? We explore questions related to three essential themes that impact on one's ability to keep the call alive. These themes are listening, community, and centeredness.

In order to perceive a call, one must maintain an attentive listening presence. This presence constitutes an ontological commitment that goes beyond the adoption of simple techniques of communication and interpersonal dynamics. By listening to our own inner voices and to the voices of others, we are able to perceive the call with greater clarity and to respond to the call with greater sensitivity and insight.

Perceiving the call necessitates a return to our authentic selves. A process of centering and decentering occurs as we come to an understanding of who we are in relation to others. The call to care, then, is lived out within community.

In reflecting on the meaning of the themes of listening, community, and centeredness, we respond to the following questions: How does the experience of listening impact on the call to care? Is it possible to be oneself and to be in community? If so, what happens when one's values and ideals are contrary to those of the community in which one is affiliated? How may spaces and places be created to nurture authenticity in community? What does it mean to be grounded or centered? How does being centered sustain the call to care? What does it mean to be decentered? What happens to a community when the familiar is made strange?

Listening and the Call to Care

The central theme of our text has been the call to care. The very nature of a call implies a primacy for the sense of hearing. A call is not so much seen as it is heard. To be called assumes that one is listening and hears the voice of God, one's inner voice, or the voice of another. The notion of listening, therefore, is of primary importance in understanding and experiencing the call to care. In this section, the notion of listening as a willful engagement of the mind is explored. The contexts in which listening may occur are articulated. The relationship between listening and language is examined. Finally, the importance of creating spaces for listening in nursing and education is addressed.

Listening as a Willful Engagement of the Mind

What does it take to listen? When is it fit to listen? To whom do we listen? Throughout our lives, we hear many voices. Voices calling to us. Voices telling us what to do. In a nursing context, we attend to our own inner voice and to the voices of patients, families, peers, and supervisors. Patients may ask to be allowed to die. Peers may ask for help in concealing a medication error. Nurse managers may ask us to remain at work for a second shift, although we are tired and fear that fatigue may impair our nursing judgments. We may ask ourselves why we ever chose to enter nursing? How do we respond to these many voices? What directs the nature of our responses?

Do we listen with the same intensity in different contexts and situations? For example, a demented patient tells us his story for the tenth time in the midst of a busy nursing unit. Do we attend to his story with the same intensity as we would a beloved friend telling us how much we have touched his or her life?

The word *listen* means to hear, to hearken, or to give ear to (Skeat 1882). In one way, listening may be thought of as a frame of mind. Listening requires a mind that is consciously, intentionally, and willfully directed to attend fully to the voice of another. At times, this frame of mind is difficult to achieve. Indeed, we are not always naturally inclined to listen. At times like these, we are guided more by a moral sense of commitment and responsibility than by a natural desire to listen.

The aim of listening is to experience communion with others. Communion is an intimate sharing characterized by contact, openness, and vulnerability and is not solely the interchange of opinion (Piles 1990). To experience communion with another requires that we listen not only to what is being said but to the context in which another is given voice.

Listening in Context

The sense of responsibility that guides the listening ear is influenced by the context in which listening occurs. What is the meaning of the relationship we have with those to whom our listening is directed? What shapes the context for listening? For example, when we listen over the telephone, we focus on the voice of the other. In person, however, we encounter another face to face. When we engage in writing, the words we convey are soundless and faceless. Yet, writing is viewed as a more formalized communicative event in society. Often, we respond with a greater sense of accountability to the written word because of the formal structure that places legal and social sanctions on our written communication.

In nursing, if an activity or event is not documented formally in the patient's legal record, it is considered never to have been done. Written documentation becomes, in large part, the legal proof of adherence to professional standards of practice. In education, our teaching is often geared to writing. Many times, speaking and listening are lived out in the context of formal presentations. Yet, true listening calls on us to be present to others in a different way.

The voice is a primary means of contact between persons. Voices carry a variety of inflections and tonal qualities that impact on the meanings that are communicated to others. Voices may be harsh, gentle, encouraging, or condescending. Often, it is the tonality of the voice that touches us. The voice creates a climate or atmosphere of its own (van Manen 1991). Meanings within speech are generated not solely by learned rules for social expression and behavior but also by genuineness of intent. When learned communication techniques are exercised devoid of genuine concern and empathy, they are often found empty and meaningless. Technique devoid of the call to care is hollow.

Voicing and Silence

Voice offers a way of knowing, communicating, and legitimating a personal, social, cultural, and political view of reality (Weiler 1988). Language, then, constitutes and legitimates a particular way of knowing. By voicing our thoughts and feelings, we make ourselves present in history and define ourselves as authors of our own life stories. Voices sound multiple subjectivities and biographies and place persons in relationship to one another through history and experience. Voices are also capable of interrogating processes that ignore or construct one's identity. In other words, through voicing, meanings are affirmed or questioned. As such, language powerfully regulates, silences, legitimates, and structures the many facets of human expression (Giroux & Freire 1988).

When voicing is seen as a metaphor for knowing, silence may be viewed as oppressive and equated with passivity or incompetence. Still, it is the interchange between voicing and listening that may allow for new ways of knowing and being to find expression. Belenky, Clinchy, Goldberger, & Tarule (1986) use the metaphor of voice to depict women's intellectual and moral development. They note that knowledge has traditionally been associated with metaphors of a visual rather than an auditory nature. For example, knowledge is often equated with "illumination," "seeing the light," or recognizing the "mind's eye." However, visual metaphors suggest distance and a separation of subject from object, as persons must stand at a distance to grasp what they are seeking to comprehend. The ear, however, suggests closeness between subject and object as persons must draw close to hear what is said and to respond. Hearing, then, implies reciprocity and dialogue. (Belenky et al., 1986).

According to Belenky et al. (1986), silence, in a sense, is a lack of awareness of the power of words to transmit knowledge. Women, in particular, may have great difficulty moving from silencing to voicing. The beginning of voicing is the development of an inner voice that recognizes and legitimates the value of one's own thoughts, feelings, and experiences. Developing an inner voice involves listening to one's own heart and adhering to an internal sense of authority. Ultimately, however, persons need to move beyond developing ways of knowing which are solely internal to nurturing a connected knowing which arises from an integration of the voices of self and others (Belenky et al. 1986).

While silence may be viewed as oppressive, it may also serve to liberate the voice of another. Indeed, speech is mediated by silence. Silence is not only the absence of speech. Silence may leave space to give another voice. This type of silence involves patience, attentive listening, and the creation of an open, trusting atmosphere. The "silence of the listening ear" is a wholehearted attentiveness to the thoughts and feelings of another. It requires a sensitivity and a knowing when to hold back one's personal views and opinions (van Manen 1991). Here, silencing is viewed as a deliberate holding back with the intent of nurturing another's thoughts and feelings to disclosure and giving another voice.

When we surrender our speech time to another, we give them a precious gift. Listening, then, is a willful surrendering. It is a sacrificial commitment to give another voice. In a sense, when we listen, we surrender our story time to another. To listen requires much energy, time, and attention. Listening is a mind occupying activity requiring great effort.

Listening as Hearkening

Levin (1989) speaks of a special kind of listening called "hearkening." Hearkening is a hearing that is moved by ontological understanding. Hearing, then, is not a static condition but a condition characterized by direction and movement. It is active and intentional.

Levin (1989) speaks of a reversal of figure and ground that takes place when we hearken. His concept of figure and ground implies differentiation. In a sense, to identify a prominent figure from its background is to differentiate between boundaries. The ground is the matrix of our Being or how we come to be who we are. It is that which defines subject and object. When we hearken, we do not so much *see* the difference between figure and ground as we *hear* the interplay between ontological differences that characterize the figure-ground dichotomy (Levin 1989).

Hearkening is not solely perceiving sounds but understanding what is perceived. With understanding comes the realization of possibilities that may develop and enrich the lives of self and others. To appropriate what we hear is to understand that what we hear makes a claim on us. Levin (1989) sees the appropriation of our hearing as a calling. We are called to respond and to make a commitment. Hearkening, then, is an authentic hearing that involves understanding of one's possibilities through reflection on Being. To hearken one must first be in tune with one's own Being. To be attuned to one's Being, one must move beyond a self-definition bounded solely by social role.

How do we listen to the inner voice of our own hearts and minds? How do we attend to the voice of our own callings?

In many ways, society has fostered the subordination of hearing to seeing and alienated the experience of listening. To cultivate hearkening, we need to restore the connection between feeling and listening. We need to cultivate a listening rooted in situatedness. This type of listening may help us to realize more fully our Being and how we are situated and contextualized. Through listening, we come to recognize our interdependence and connectedness with others. We are a part of a matrix of intertwined identities, differences, and destinies. Hearkening, then, presupposes an ethics of relatedness, care, and responsibility (Levin 1989).

As persons called to care, we need to develop a capacity for hearkening. Hearkening is a desiring to hear. It is making hearing possible, and it is being open to what is heard. Persons seeking to hearken need to remain open and aware of the surrounding field in which their listening and voicing are embedded (Levin 1989).

When we hearken, we also listen into the silence. In other words, we remain open to silence. Silence is a listening openness. To hear something, we give it our silence. It is difficult to cultivate silence in our present day. Nurturing silence requires calmness, relaxation, and a well-balanced state of body and mind (Levin, 1989). All of these conditions are antithetical to nursing and educational milieus. However, the very nature of listening is playful, and it demands a tolerance for wandering, drifting, and openness. Levin (1989) refers to this type of listening as "vagabond listening." Vagabond listening requires an acceptance of uncertainty of where the conversation will lead.

Listening as a Hermeneutic Process

Hearkening is characterized by opening, laying out, and gathering in (Levin, 1989). Like the hermeneutic spiral, being open to feelings, laying out one's history, and gathering in that which the other brings to us has an echoic dimension. Levin (1989) identifies the echo as the essence of things. Echoing implies an understanding of the full measure or substance of an entity. The echo is deconstructive. It sets up vibrations of uncertainty. It challenges existing assumptions. The echo teaches the presence of absence and the absence of presence. In other words, what we believe to be true and present is called into question and what we are not consciously aware of, that is, what is absent from our perceived reality, is brought to disclosure. Through the echo, the presence of the grounding of one's life experiences and historical conditions that shape one's present questions and situations becomes audible (Levin 1989).

Hearing as a gathering in implies acceptance, attention, and response to what is heard. We need to extend the reach of our listening to be able to gather in more. For example, by listening in diverse contexts, we expand our listening boundaries. To listen in diversity requires a suspending of our prejudices, likes, and dislikes in order to allow what is there to speak. A gathering in, in this sense, is not a grasping, fixating gesture but an openness to receive what is outside of us (Levin 1989).

This type of listening means that we experience time differently. There is an interplay of past, present, and future gathered into the present moment. This interplay moves us away from the conventional linear conception of time and opens our awareness to the dimension of time as a whole (Levin, 1989).

The history of Western civilization was originally passed down through the oral tradition. Hearing belonged to history. Nursing is also steeped in an oral tradition (Street 1992), as Levin indicates: "When

I listen to myself, to my words, to the sound of my voice, I can hear others; I hear others 'inside' myself...Conversely, when I listen to others, I can hear myself...We resonate and echo one another. I can hear my ancestors: their absence is present, their presence is the presence of an echo, an audible absence" (Levin 1989, p. 272). In this passage, Levin describes the echo of the voices of history brought into the present. Through hearing, we see how our identities and destinies are intertwined with others. By retrieving this sense of intertwining, we may assume responsibility for others by seeing their interconnectedness with us.

Language and Listening

Speech is the proclamation of reciprocity between persons (Buber 1973). Language could not exist without address. Dialogue came before monologue. Language arose out of partnership. "Even when in a solitude beyond the range of call, the hearerless word pressed against the throat, this word was connected with the primal possibility, that of being heard" (Glatzer 1966, p. 103). Therefore speaking and listening presuppose relationship and partnership. With acceptance of another as a partner in dialogue comes affirmation of him or her as a person (Glatzer 1966).

It is by listening that we are gathered into compassion. Therefore, our range of compassion is dependent on our listening skill. To listen well requires avoidance of distraction as well as concentrated attention, silence, patience, and time. There is also a "staying with" dimension needed to listen long enough to develop familiarity and intimacy to what is being heard (Levin 1989). By making spaces for listening, we nurture this sense of relationship and responsibility and engage in what is truly an ethical and moral practice.

Creating Spaces for Listening and Voicing

Nursing and education have adopted the language of the behavioral sciences to give their professions voice. This type of language, while allowing for precision in measurement and objectification of behavior, does not seem to capture adequately the major thrust of both nursing and education; that is, the call to care for others. What is needed is a language that allows one to speak more directly about the fundamental nature of what it means to be called to care. Would it be possible to develop a language that is more personal and more richly captures the feelings, thoughts, and ideas inherent in the notion of a call? Such a language would need to be able to express the personal meanings that are brought to words and the historical and social context in which our language and communication practices unfold.

Regardless of the language used to communicate, a tension inevitably exists as we contemplate what is excluded from language and what language is unable to communicate fully. All language, in some way, can become alienating and exclusive. Language is incomplete unless it occurs with the recipient sense of listening needed to appreciate and understand the nature of our very Being that is called forth through language. Regardless of the language we use, we have to ask ourselves whether we are trying to dominate others through the model of our language. What is the intent behind our communications?

How do we create spaces to nurture listening and voicing? In nursing, the language used to communicate is highly technical and tends to have meaning only to those in the profession. By professionalizing our language in this way, we alienate and exclude the recipients of our care from entering into our conversations. These are persons with whom we share the call to care. In some way, these are the persons who have called us to care. How can we invite them back into the conversation? Conversely, how may we reenter their conversation from which we ourselves have become alienated?

By bringing a narrative story structure to our language, we may open our conversation to others and move away from words and expressions that have meaning only to those in the profession. Perhaps what is needed is to nurture a more personal language within the profession. This language would make valid and legitimate such terms as *love, humility, vulnerability, and authenticity.*

To increase one's own and other's sensitivity to the power of words, it may be helpful to explore with students what meaning they bring to words. First semester students may be given a list of professional jargon and asked to reflect on the personal meaning of these terms. What would it be like to hear these words as a patient? Reflections on this activity may be saved until the end of the program. How have the students perceptions changed over time? Students may also be encouraged to trace the etymology of words and professional terms. In what way have the meaning of words been hidden and/or distorted from their original use?

Building community means taking the time to listen to other's stories. Stories shape who we are and make us unique (Huebner 1987). To provide spaces for listening and voicing, it is important to nurture interpersonal dialogue (oral and written)—between student and patient, student and teacher, student and student, and teacher and patient— that reflects and encourages the sharing of life stories.

Students may need to practice using their sense of listening. How does one incorporate listening experiences into the curriculum? It may be helpful to consider using student text as a basis for listening and responding. Tape recording or videotaping group conferences, discussions, or nurse-patient interactions may serve as a point of departure for reflection and dialogue. Listening exercises may be conducted through reflection on selected taped conversations and events. The videotape may be viewed without sound. Discussion may ensue regarding whether it is possible to separate seeing from listening. What is lost or gained in the process? How are our sensibilities awakened differently when we listen versus watch? What feelings and ideas emerge from watching a videotape without sound or from listening to an audiotape without seeing the persons engaged in dialogue?

Students may also engage in experiences with the hearing and visually impaired. What sounds and senses are magnified or dulled? Sounds common in a nursing practice setting may be taped and played to students. Sounds have a way of penetrating through the body. We can turn away our faces to avoid seeing painful sights. It is easier to divert our eyes than our ears. What are students responses to sounds of death, pain, birth, or tears? What would it be like for a patient to hear the sounds of doctors whispering outside one's room? What is it like to hear the sound of nasogastric suctioning, of a ventilator in an intensive care unit, or of a door locking shut on a psychiatric ward? What meanings do these sounds have for persons who are guests in the health care setting?

How does one's presence impact on the sounds of nursing? Students may listen to tapes of a comforting soothing voice, a voice of gratitude, a voice of refusal of care, or a voice of dissatisfaction with inattentive care. Students may be asked to share stories or encourage patients, peers, or others to tell their stories of meaningful caring experiences. Attention may be directed to not only what is said but to voice tone and intensity and visual expressions and to the personal feelings that listening to other's stories engenders.

How is hearkening made a norm? How may one create an environment where communion is valued? Ultimately, listening should be legitimated as a valued and necessary part of one's caregiving practice. For example, listening should be considered in making patient assignments and should be written into the formal nursing care plan as a valid and legitimate therapeutic intervention. In addition, persons may be encouraged to listen to their own inner voices by sharing and reflecting on their own personal calls to care and the historical and social contexts that shape their life choices and commitments. By encouraging self-reflection and by nurturing interpersonal dialogue that give voice to the sharing of life stories, one may come to realize more fully the context in which one's call to care is perceived, responded to, and lived out.

Listening is a willful engagement of the mind with the intent of experiencing communion with others. Listening is affected by the context in which one is called to listen and to respond. Speech and language are deeply tied to the listening experience. Language would not be possible without the hope of being heard. It is by listening that we are gathered into compassion for others. By creating spaces for listening and hearkening in professional practice, the call to care may be realized, valued, sustained, and appreciated more fully. Since the call to care is lived out within community, one is challenged to hearken to the common values and ideals represented by being in a community, while, at the same time, allowing the voices of diversity within a community to find expression.

Creating Conversational Communities

A context for listening and centering may be a spontaneous meeting of friends and companions, or it could be a deliberate gathering of persons committed to creating a different way of being with one another. As participants in a conversational community individuals come with a strong sense of themselves and their own independence, yet are committed to creating a true community—a reflective, listening, conversational "we." Furthermore, the community is viewed not as an end in itself but rather as a power-sharing way of being with others in genuine conversation, reflective thought, and deliberate action. Conversation, thought, and action are directed toward fostering authentic connections among members as well as personal and social transformation around valued issues of mutual concern. This community respects difference and diversity while it works toward equalizing power and empowerment.

What would the lived experience be like in such a community? What would it be like to experience the power of connection—of-being-with—not the power-over of domination? How would one's individualism and independence be limited in a community that honors connectedness? How might we as educators and nurses establish communities to advance shared views as we work toward creating possibilities for the future?

Joining communities of reflection, conversation, and action is one way of developing authentic connections among persons with shared interests and concerns. Such an experience offers an opportunity to decrease one's isolation, and the outcome has the potential for leading to personal growth and transformation.

Power Relations in Conversational Communities

Groups also serve as a powerful basis for movement and the betterment of the common good. Wheeler and Chinn, in *Peace and Power: A Handbook of Feminist Process*, call us to rethink how we approach group interactions and what we intend or hope to accomplish. Drawing on ideas of peace, praxis, and empowerment, they challenge us to create new realities for nurturing each other and being together.

Changing the intent and process of a community is the equivalent of renaming a part of our world. Beittel with Beittel (1991) asserts that renaming and adding new qualities to that which is named is a way of becoming involved in the politics of things. They suggest that renaming moves us "away from the tired humanism toward a new poetic Genesis where the world again acts as a nurturant mother. Spirit and matter meet. The ends of the chain join" (p. 80).

How does one tap the reality of power in ways that empower those who may feel powerless? How can our world again be a nurturant mother? How can we step outside our usual power-devouring situatedness to be regenerated? What is concealed and revealed in our "inheritance" that might open possibilities for a different and better future?

We can no longer allow power to be something "out there" rather then a process we all may share. Such thinking undermines our own ability to make a difference. If we are to make transformational changes in nursing education and practice, we must have a fuller understanding of our individual capabilities and the power of connection and collectivity. Kriesberg (1992) notes that "empowerment does not assume control of resisting others, but emerges from work with others who are also deciding, acting, and making a difference" (p. xi). This sense of empowerment requires an exploration of the differences between "power-over," "power-with," and "power-from-within."

A shift in our thinking from power-over to power-with relations in a community would be radical. It would involve seeing power as a process we participate in and as shared ownership of the community. Community ownership and power would not be exerted over members. The challenge then becomes one of developing one's own personal power (power-from-within) and learning how to be in community (power-with) with those who choose to respond to our invitation and are committed to shared projects. "In this type of power, strength does not mean the ability to impose one's will on another [power-over] rather,

TABLE 11.1

Characteristics of "With-ness"

Being-with Others	Being over, under, or away from Others
Spontaneity, lives in the moment	Use of methods and techniques, out of touch with present moment, responds to past or future
Available, open, feels with	Tuned out, closed, analytical
Emergent relationships, being personal	Prescribed relationships, being in role, interpersonal distancing
Present, intimate	Aloof, withdrawn, separate
Questions the present and the status quo	Reinforces the past, invests in the status quo
Allows self and others to be, enjoys diversity and change	Controls self and others, makes demands
Synergistic action, doing with	Role-bound action, dominance, or submission
Strength from connection	Strength from cohesion and resistance
Power from entering in relation	Power from domination

M. T. Neal, "Preceptorship and Mentoring in Psychiatric Nursing," (Paper presented at Psychiatric Nursing Grand Rounds, University of Maryland Medical System, Baltimore, September 1992).

strength is expressed in openness to other voices, openness to change and innovation, and trust in the growth that comes as people work together" (Kreisberg 1992, p. xii). Strength evolves from knowing why we choose to stand together. (For a comparison of characteristics of "with-ness," see table 11.1.)

From a curricular perspective, being-with students implies providing a student-focused course of study with many aspects being mutually generated (Hultgren 1992). All knowing/learning would be valued and epiphanies would be a frequent pleasure. Faculty and students would work toward an evolving, shared vision of thought and action. Interactions would be caring and nurturing as well as challenging and transformative. Students and teachers would see each other as allies or partners. The focus would be on the accomplishment of learning and on personal transformation growing out of the shared experiences.

In contrast, a curriculum that exerts power-over students would be more teacher controlled with prescribed and measurable outcomes. The teachers would select the content and define the product. Learning activities would be teacher planned and initiated. The focus would be on the student as product of the curriculum as defined on paper.

Facing Each Other as Equals—"Power-With"

Thoughts and actions grow out of developing a self-consciousness around shared moral concerns. When this happens we face each other in the authenticity of our actual being. Also implied by the process is the valuing of authenticity and uniqueness along with bonds of connection. One would not expect to find the absence of difference. Rather, meeting others from diverse backgrounds and points of view is essential for growth and transformation. Difference and disagreement are what conversation is about in the quest for truth. It is out of the dialectic of disagreement that something new can emerge. It is therefore instructive to seek out resistance and difference, along with support and affirmation, if real progress is to be made.

Enmeshed in the notion of being-with is a commitment to a life of dialogue—an ongoing conversation involving listening and speaking, the use of voice to give language and to share commonality of meaning. Being-with others in conversation is both a present happening as well as an ongoing process or movement. It is a dialogic process by which we understand, change, and gather the fullness of life's offerings.

Waking Up to "Power-From-Within"

Wheeler and Chinn (1989) define empowerment as "growth of personal strength, power and ability to enact one's will and love for Self in the context of love for others" (p. 2). Empowerment is not self-indulgent. It is strength that emerges from inward listening as well as intentional listening to others. When we no longer listen to and express our visions and imagination, our world begins to shrink and our personal power is diminished. How then might we open a space in the curriculum for vision-centered interactions and realities? How might we use our imagination in the service of creating new possibilities and in bettering our world? Paying attention to listening—that is, inner listening to one's soul or listening in dialogue—is important for self and for life in community. Listening to messages from within inspires, directs, and makes audible expression of our inner world: inner listening empowers.

We are talking here about simultaneous listening and speaking, listening not so much as a function of the ear but as an act of inner receptivity where the whole person hears. It may be the skin that prickles or the muscles that tense—to silence, to sound, to chaos, to pain, to dreams, to imagination. How can we learn to listen and then respond to this inner listening, which allows a different form of language to be? How can we allow our dreams, fantasies, desires, and imaginations to come into our listening? How can we be open to what we hear, open to what we then must say, and empowered from the saying?

Part of the answer lives in experience and the other in meaning. Through experiences such as centering or imagery one gains access to inner pictures and sounds; from them one takes meaning. How much authority do we give this invisible inner voice? How can the structure of a conversational community provide the audience for one's inner listening in a way which sustains life, inner unity, centeredness, and empowerment? Thinking about centering and imagining leads to wondering how one might stay centered and engage one's internal power. Richards (1962) in describing her work with making clay vessels, asserts that we must be passionate and be able to Be. "We must be able to let the intensity—the Dionysian rapture and disorder and the celebration of chaos, of potentiality, the experience of surrender—...live in our bodies, in our hands, through our hands into the materials we work with" (p. 12). From these experiences we advance self-knowledge and our knowing of the world. How might being in community give one the courage to Be? What kind of Being in today's world is required for transformation?

Imagining New Forms of Human Relationships

Moccia (1990) urges nurse educators to reclaim our communities and create a new reality for education and practice. Arguing for a redefinition of ourselves and our institutions that is grounded in caring values, she challenges nurses to develop a collective voice and the use of power in rebuilding communities and in "reclaiming spaces and places for humane and caring interactions, and of articulating a compelling vision of another way for society and its people to be" (p. 74).

What is needed to make such a challenge real? Buber (1961) asserts that "community is the being no longer side by side (and, one might add, above and below) but *with* one another of a multitude of persons. And this multitude, though it moves towards one goal, yet experiences everywhere a turning to, a dynamic facing of, the others, a flowing from *I* to *Thou*. Community is where community happens" (p. 51). He describes a "happening" as a group that arises out of mutuality—the "essential *we*." He says, "Only when I have to do with another essentially, that is, in such a way that he is no longer a phenomenon of my *I*, but instead is my *Thou*, do I experience reality of speech with another—in the irrefragable genuineness of mutuality" (p. 72). For Buber, real living is meeting (1958, p. 11). What would make our meetings into transforming "we" encounters? How might our living be made authentically real through community? What betterment would result?

Centeredness is Central to Keeping the Call Alive

A Being centered receives ongoing nourishment and energy to continue to strengthen self and reach out to community. Centering can be described as a returning home, a sense of place to come back to, finding comfort in renewed self-awareness, and in hearing a call for response to greater human need beyond oneself. Centering means being authentic, more whole, creative, and free. From the aesthetic sense, in drawing from the arts, centeredness is a theme that impacts on keeping the call alive. "When on center, the self feels different: one feels warm, *on rayonne*, in touch, the power of life a substance like an air in which one lives and has one's being with all other things, drinking it in and giving it off, at the same time quiet and at rest within it" (Richards 1964, p. 56).

Centeredness implies growth. Growth is possible, a movement to and fro, a movement beyond one's grounding, a reaching out to others in response to a call to care. In the process of growing, of ascending and becoming more, one is surrounded by a larger circle of community, bounded but not confined.

Being at Home with Self and Others

Van Manen (1984) postulates that in the calling one may find "being" (p. 155). The call is described as silent, as conscience coming from within self, attuned by anxiety concerning its potential for being. A call to conscience summons the self to be all it can be through care. The calling of self to itself summons a return from lostness and reflects concern for others (Heidegger 1962, p. 322). Mayerhoff comments: "Through caring for certain others, by serving them through caring, a man lives the meaning of his own life. In the sense in which a man can ever be said to be at home in the world, he is at home not through dominating or explaining or appreciating, but through caring and being cared for" (Mayeroff 1971, p. 2).

In being centered, a person is able to be at home through caring and being cared for. In caring, a process for helping another grow and actualize, the one cared for is experienced as an extension of self. Growth of the other person is tied into one's own sense of well-being. Through helping another grow, the self is actualized (Mayeroff 1971, p. 22).

As an axle forms the center of a wheel and joins circles together, persons joined together in care may be connected through an inner core or center of being. Care forms the axle or link among persons and a sense of comfort evolves as centers are strengthened. A sense of empowerment is also experienced as centered persons come together with a common focus.

It is the center of a wheel that allows movement—the inner space. Persons may journey together sharing face to face or joined side by side. A balance is easier to maintain when persons are psychologically joined through a common core. Being is the center core of personhood. Persons unite at the level of Being and extend themselves to enact activities of knowing and doing in response to a call to care.

In everyday tasks we may become lost in an array of differing values and personal understandings. In going astray we may lose sight of new possibilities for caring. We may return home for renewal, a caring for self, a time for reflection and healing. Finding the way home or centering to become replenished means following a strong signal of purpose for self and one's being in the world. We take many turns during our adventure in life and we may find that "the power of self is its self centeredness or self awareness" (Tillich 1954).

Spirituality

What does it mean to be centered or grounded and how does being centered sustain the call to care? Centering means finding hope and peace and preparing anew to hear and respond to a call to care. A spiritual sense or a commitment to something larger than self may guide one to respond to a call in a very profound way. Spiritual insights may bring an inner order. "We are spiritual beings by nature, but we also have a physical body and a mind. This triune nature—body, mind and spirit—reflects the image of God. We are given the capacity to think, to create, to love, to care about and for, and to be compassionate" (Carson 1993, p. 25).

The following description of a caring physician is a story of a person being centered in a spiritual sense.[1] The physician seemed to understand the meaning of his own life and thus could be more fully present and make a difference in the lives of others.

A newspaper story about the physician described him as kind and humble giving tirelessly of self to others. He is remembered as one who was constantly concerned for those who were burdened by troubles and adversity. He seemed to know when others were in need whether they were his patients, their families, or members of the staff. It was written that he was revered and devoted to family, medicine, and a deep spiritual faith. It was the sense of a greater power that seemed to guide him. "Once when praised for his talents as a surgeon, . . . [he] blushed and said that if he had any abilities, it was only because he was an instrument of a divine hand" (Springer 1991, p. A8). Those in his care said that his spirituality and warm bedside manner provided great comfort. He was able to convey a sense that "life was more than just now." "His was a deep and abiding faith that was at the forefront of everything he did. It nourished and sustained him in his daily life" (DeVine 1991).

Joy in living and joy in doing for others is central to being and reflects a caring being. In describing another person who made a difference, Chet, a twelve-year-old, was said to radiate a smile that was "a witness to the happiness that filled his being." His joy in doing for others "testified to the love and genuine concern he felt for other people" (White 1981). Life was lived beautifully, completely, and with love and that life inspired others to live life more joyfully and more beautifully. In being involved in joyful acts, awareness of self seems to disappear, but the sense of self emerges stronger after an experience. A process of centering and decentering occurs as we come to understand who we are in relation to others.

These stories are about persons who made a difference in the lives of others. These are persons who are remembered as compassionate and loving. They appear selfless. However, at their core there is a strong sense of self that elicits strength and makes movement toward people possible. In finding self, one is transformed. We are awakened to responsibility of other "by bringing into center all the elements of our sensations and our thinking and our emotions and our will: all the realities of our bodies and our souls" (Richards 1964, p. 36). In a spiritual sense we are called "out of darkness into his marvelous light" (1 Peter 2:9).

As nurses we are called to acknowledge our spiritual journey, "for it is in the continuous meeting of one's own spiritual needs that one will know the meaning of spiritual well-being" (Stoll 1989, p. 21). Attentiveness to spiritual needs is caring in a very profound sense.

One nurse described her feeling of spirituality in nursing as: "A deep sense of ministration to the individual. You minister to the spirit within the body. Sometimes you will not even recognize the person outwardly because of the deterioration. You minister to the spirit" (Montgomery 1992, p. 46).

The nurse is able to connect with the spirit of the patient even when the person may be unable to communicate in response. "The spiritual nature of the connection also serves as an important resource from which the caregiver can derive meaning that sustain him or her through loss and other stressors associated with caring" (Montgomery 1992, p. 50).

Freedom to Be

In spiritual transcendence we are released from isolation and are free to unite with others, transcending to greater meaning in relationships (Montgomery 1992). Carson (1993) describes spirituality as having both vertical and horizontal dimensions; the horizontal deal with self, others and the environment whereas the vertical dimension is in relationship to God. "Because of the transforming action of God on our spirits, spiritual growth defies being boxed in to conform to a neat, sequential stage theory" (Carson 1993, p. 26).

We make choices all the time, meaning we are free to become, to experience ongoing growth, and sustain a call to care. Striving and hoping are inherent in our centeredness, and when we feel in control or in balance, "we feel a sense of exhilaration, a deep sense of enjoyment" (Csikszentmihalyi 1990, p. 3). Arnold (1989) described spirituality as "an extraordinary union with a sacred energy that reaches beyond ordinary knowledge of the everyday world to embody the ultimate virtues of life in the form of hope, courage, faith, honor, love, acceptance, and meaningful encounter with death (p. 322).

Being centered means sensing both self-awareness and a responsibility to one's community. There is a synergy or balance with the environment and the focus is toward living harmoniously (Csikszentmihalyi 1990). Living harmoniously is living responsibly with a sense of spontaneity. Centering is a means to live life as an art—that is a "mode of being in which elements of form and content; style and meaning; feeling and rhythm—all the living perception may be imaged forth in a way that does not sacrifice the moving character of the world" (Richards 1964, p. 40). In bringing self into a centering mode, we bring it into a union with other elements. This is love for others.

When we join with others we become in a way decentered. In the process of our dissertation research we were engaged in decentering as we became transformed in the process of becoming recentered. A metamorphosis of who we are and how we are with others became evident, and we continue to ask, What does it mean to be centered, to be decentered and to be recentered? Are these all parts that sustain the call to care and help us to live our lives in meaningful ways? How does being together and creating meanings influence our development as persons? What would others see in us as we live out caring in community?

The call, the hearing of the call, and the sustainment of the call have a spiritual component to them. We are called to care for one another and to be with others as we would like them to be with us. To care for others we need to move outward from a firm foundation, to build on prior learning and move beyond. A spiritual sense may provide the energy for the inner strength. "In order to be there for others, we also bring a real need to be rooted in sources that nourish and animate the spirit of our being" (Karl 1992, p. 10).

Note

1. Two personal encounters had relevance for this chapter. The physician mentioned in this text is the brother of one of the authors, Emily Slunt. He died during the writing of the book. Chet was a neighbor who was adored by both children and adults alike.

References

Arnold, E. (1989). Burnout as a spiritual issue: Rediscovering meaning in nursing practice. In V. B. Carson, *Spiritual dimensions of nursing practice* (pp. 320–53) Philadelphia: W. B. Sanders Company.

Beittel, K., with Beittel, J. (1991). *A celebration of art and consciousness*. State College, PA: Happy Valley Healing Arts.

Belenky, M., Clinchy, B., Goldberger, N., & Tarule, J. (1986). *Women's ways of knowing: The development of self, voice and mind*. New York: Basic Books.

Buber, M. L. (1961). *Between man and man*. (R. G. Smith, Trans.). London: Fontana Library. (Original work published 1947)

Buber, M. L. (1968). *I and thou*. (R. G. Smith, Trans.). New York: Scribner's.

Buber, M. L. (1973). *Meetings*. LaSalle, IL: Open Court.

Carson, V. B. (1993) Spirituality: Generic or Christian? *Journal of Christian Nursing*, Winter, 24–7.

Csikszentmihalyi, M. (1990). *Flow.* New York: HarperCollins.

Devine, T. (1991, July 14). Dr. Dave Todd: His death leaves a void. *The Forum,* p. 21.

Giroux, H., & Freire, P. (1988). Preface. In K. Weiler (Ed.), *Women teaching for change: Gender, class, and power* (pp. ix–xiv). Boston: Bergin & Garvey.

Glatzer, N. (Ed.). (1966). *The way of response: Martin Buber.* New York: Schocken Books.

Heidegger, M. (1962). *Being and time.* (J. Macquarrie & E. Robinson, Trans.). New York: Harper & Row. (Original work published 1927)

Huebner, D. (1987). The vocation of teaching. In F. S. Bolin & J. M. Falk (Eds.), *Teacher renewal: Professional issues, personal choices* (pp. 17–29). New York: Teachers College Press.

Hultgren, F. H. (1992). The transformative power of "being with" students in teaching. In L. Peterat & E. Vaines (Eds.), *Lives and plans: Signs for transforming practice* (pp. 221–42). Mission Hills, CA: Glenco Division, Macmillan McGraw-Hill.

Karl, J. (1992). Being there: Who do you bring to practice? In D. Gaut (Ed.), *The presence of caring in nursing* (pp. 1–13). New York: National League for Nursing.

Kreisberg, S. (1992). *Transforming power: Domination, empowerment, and education.* Albany: State University of New York Press.

Levin, D. M. (1989). *The listening self: Personal growth, social change and the closure of metaphysics.* New York: Routledge.

Mayeroff, M. (1971). *On caring.* New York: Harper & Row.

Moccia, P. (1990). Re-claiming our communities. *Nursing Outlook, 38*(20), 73–6.

Montgomery, C. (1992). The spiritual connection: Nurses' perceptions of the experience of caring. In D. Gaut (Ed.). *The presence of caring in nursing* (pp. 39–52). New York: National League for Nursing.

Neal, M. T. (1992, September). *Preceptorship and mentoring in psychiatric nursing.* Paper presented at Psychiatric Nursing Grand Rounds, University of Maryland Medical System, Baltimore.

Piles, C. (1990). Communion: A vital link in the process of conveying love, trust, and forgiveness. In R. Stoll (Ed.), *Concepts in nursing: A Christian perspective* (pp. 71-86). Madison: Intervarsity Christian Fellowship.

Richards, M. C. (1964). *Centering in pottery, poetry, and the person.* Middletown, CT: Wesleyan University Press. (Original work published 1962)

Skeat, W. (1882). *An etymological dictionary of the English language.* Oxford: Clarendon Press.

Springer, P. (1991, July, 13). Doctor remembered for caring attitude. *The Forum,* pp. A1, A8.

Stoll, R. (1989). The essence of spirituality. In V. B. Carson, *Spiritual dimensions of nursing practice* (pp. 4–23). Philadelphia: W. B. Saunders Company.

Street, A. F. (1992). *Inside nursing: A critical ethnography of clinical nursing practice.* Albany: State University of New York Press.

Tillich, P. (1954). *Love, power, and justice.* London: Oxford University Press.

van Manen, M. (1984). Reflections on teacher competence and pedagogic competence. In E. Short (Ed.), *Competence: Inquiries into its meaning and acquisition in educational settings* (pp. 141–58). Lanham, MD: University Press of America.

van Manen, M. (1991). *The tact of teaching.* Albany: State University of New York Press.

Weiler, K. (1988). *Women teaching for change: Gender, class, and power.* Boston: Bergin & Garvey.

Wheeler, C. E., & Chinn, P. L. (1989). *Peace and power: A handbook of feminist process.* New York: National League for Nursing.

White, T. (1981). The meditation for Chet's memorial service. Burtonsville, MD: Epiphany Lutheran Church.

Index